Notes on MJT

(Forensic Medicine & Toxicology)

By

Dr. Debasish Kundu Ph.D.

Assisted By

Dr. Ravi Justin Raj

NMD, LLB

Edited By

Dr. Malik A.K. Awan

B.S., M.S. (Psychology), D.C.L., D.D. (U.S.A.), Ph.D. (London)

Originals

Delhi

First Published 2017

Illustrations: Prof. Dr. Debasish Kundu

ISBN 13: 978-81-8454-190-8

ISBN 10: 81-8454-190-2

Published By

Originals

A-6, Second Floor, Nimri Commercial Centre,

Ashok Vihar Phase-4, Delhi - 110 052 (India)

Tel.: +91 11 2730 2453 Fax: 011 4706 1936

Website: www.Lppindia.com, e-mail: info@Lppindia.com

Printed At

D K Fine Art Press P Ltd.

Delhi-110052

PRINTED IN INDIA

DEDICATION

To my son Aditya

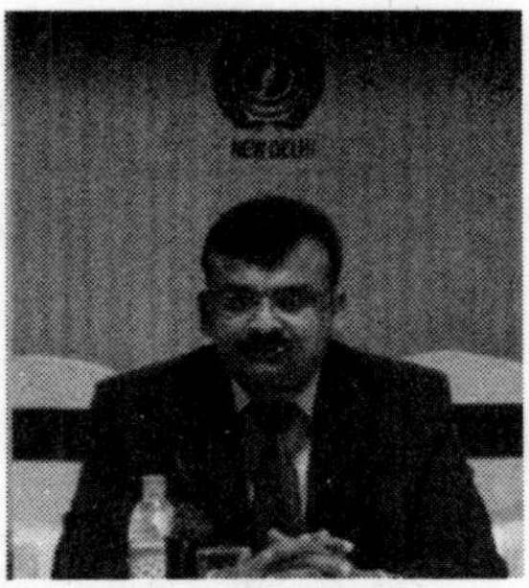

Foreword

I am pleased to have the opportunity to write foreword for the book of Notes on MJT (Forensic Medicine and Toxicology) which is written by Dr. Debasish Kundu for ADEH students. Because I have a dream for all my Electro Homoeopathic practitioners that one day they must get an official Certificate from any Government Agency and I am happy to say that Maharashtra is the First State in India to offer an Official Electro Homoeopathy Certificate which is being awarded by the Government Agency. Also I have some friends who helped me to fulfill my dream to introduce a Government recognised ADVANCE DIPLOMA IN ELECTRO HOMOEOPATHY (ADEH) course in Maharashtra.

When word comes "ADVANCED" means something new and scientific, so while reading the contents of the book, I found something new and advanced. Since long time Dr. Kundu is writing books on different subjects which are very easy to understand and rich in contents, so I believe this book will help all the Students, Practitioners & Lovers of Electro-Homoeopathy besides students in perusing ADEH examination which contains the study material mentioned in Syllabus by MSBVE, Mumbai. This entire course material will help to improve the knowledge in Electro Homoeopathy subject.

Dr. Trideep Guha
BPTH, MD (ECH) MBA, Ph.D., MRCE (USA)
Chairman
Educational & Medical/Paramedical Council of India
Executive Member:
Paramedical Syllabus Committee,
MSBVEE, Mumbai (Govt. of Maharashtra)

Email id
drtrideep.g@gmail.com, empci@hotmail.com
Visit us at :
www.empci.com

Published By

Originals

A-6, Second Floor, Nimri Commercial Centre,
Ashok Vihar Phase-4, Delhi - 110 052 (India)
Tel.: +91 11 2730 2453 Fax: 011 4706 1936
Website: www.Lppindia.com
e-mail: info@Lppindia.com

In Association with

ADEH PRACTISIONERS ASSOCIATION MAHARASHTRA

N-123, Second floor, Infront of Devanjali flats,
Reshimbag, City & District : Nagpur
State : Maharashtra Country : INDIA
Phone : +91-712-2700606, +91-712-2700651, +91-712-2700777

Contents

Part I
Forensic Medicine

Part II

Toxicology

Preface

Medical jurisprudence is a science of applying medical facts to legal problems. Forensic medicine and Toxicology are the most important areas of Medical Jurisprudence. Forensic Medicine is often considered to be a vital instrument for the detection or investigation of crime and the administration of justice, providing crucial information about the evidence found at crime scene, where the knowledge of the methodologies or clinical trials of the substances are used in the investigation of a crime where the examination is done in the laboratories about the causes or injury of the death. Toxicology derives from the Ancient Greek word 'Toxicos' which means toxic or poisonous. It is the branch of medicine that deals with the harmful effects of various chemicals on living beings or organisms.

Authors hope to cater to the needs of students and professionals in this field with concise yet updated and descriptive information encompassing all aspects related to Forensic Medicine and Toxicology.

Dr. Debasish Kundu

Dr. Ravi Justin Raj

Part I
Forensic Medicine

1

Introduction

Medical Jurisprudence is the branch of medicine that deals with the application of medical knowledge to the purpose of law and in the administration of justice. It is the application of the basic clinical, medical paramedical and toxicological sciences to elucidate forensic matters.

Originally the terms forensic medicine and medical jurisprudence are synonymous, and in common practice are used interchangeably in relation with the practice of medico-legal profession.

On the other hand, medical jurisprudence, or forensic science and toxicology, denotes knowledge of law in relation to the practice of medicine. It concerns with the study of the right, duties and obligations of medical practitioner with particular reference to those arising from doctor-patient relationship. This is provided by the Code of Ethics of Medical Profession.

Scope of Forensic Medicine

The Scope of Forensic Medicine is quite broad and encompassing. It is the application of medical and paramedical sciences as demanded by law and administration of justice. The knowledge of the nature and extent of wounds had been acquired in surgery, abortion in gynecology, sudden death and effect of trauma in pathology, etc., aside from having knowledge of the basic medical sciences, like anatomy, physiology, biochemistry, physics and other allied sciences.

It is concerned with a broad range of medical, legal and ethical issues, as well as human rights and rights of individuals.

The medico legal officers have a duty to act in their patients best interest and can be charged in a court of law if they fail to do so. On the other hand, he or she may be required to act in the interest of third parties if his patient is in danger to others. Failure to do so many lead to legal action against the said medical officers.

The medico-legal officers assessed injured individuals and the degree of impairment they cause. This allows courts to determine and award damages. They may also be required to assess the mental status of accused persons and whether they are fit to stand trial. They may also determine whether an individual is of sound mind and capable of getting into a binding contract with another party.

Ordinary Physician vs. Forensic Doctor

Hereunder are some of the important distinctions between an ordinary physician and forensic doctor, as follows:

1. An ordinary physician examines the point of view of treatment while the forensic doctor sees injury or disease on the point of view of cause.
2. The purpose of an ordinary physician in the examination of a patient is to arrive at a definite diagnosis to that appropriate treatment can be instituted, while the purpose of the medical-jurist in the examination of a patient is to include bodily lesions in his reports and testify before the court or before an investigative body, thus giving justice to whom it is due.
3. Minor or trivial injuries are usually ignored by an ordinary physician in as much as they do not require usual treatment, while the medical jurists must record all bodily injuries even if they are small or minor, because these injuries may be proofs to qualify the crime or to justify the act.

Areas of Forensic Medicine

Hereunder are the different areas that commonly involved in forensic medicine are as follows:

1. Anatomy

It is a branch of biology and medicine that is the consideration of the structure of living things. It is a general term that includes human anatomy, animal anatomy, and plant anatomy. In some of its facets anatomy is closely related to embryology, comparative anatomy and comparative embryology, through common roots in evolution.

2. Pathology

It is the precise study and diagnosis of disease. The word pathology is from Ancient Green pathos, feeling, suffering and logia, the study of, which refers to the process of defining a condition or behavior as pathological, e.g. pathological gambling. Pathology is synonymous with diseases.

3. Psychiatry

It is the medical specialty devoted to the study and treatment of mental disorders. These mental disorders include various affective, behavioral, cognitive and perceptual abnormalities, and which literally means the medical treatment of the mind. A medical doctor specializing in psychiatry is a psychiatrist.

Brief History of Medical Jurisprudence

The 'art of healing' began thousands of years ago with the innovations of the primitive man trying to provide relief to those close to him, in sickness and suffering, motivated by feelings of sympathy and kindness.

In the absence of an obvious explanation, his limited intelligence attributed disease and other calamities to the anger of God, the invasion of the body by evil spirits or the influence of stars and planets.

As a logical sequence, the medicine then practiced consisted in appeasing God by prayers and rituals and sacrifices, driving out evil spirits from the human body.

There is also evidence that prehistoric man improvised stone and flint instruments with which he performed circumcisions, amputations and trephining of skulls.

It is thus obvious that medicine in the prehistoric era (5000 BC) was intermingled with superstition, religion, magic and witchcraft.

Elements of prehistoric medicine are still present in many countries.

Primitive man may be extinct, but the supernatural theory of disease in which he believed is not yet extinct in our modern society.

Indian Medicine

Indian medicine is as ancient as Hindu Civilisation. Ayurveda by definition implies 'The Science of Life'. (Ayurveda is a Sanskrit word derived from two roots: Ayur, which means life, and Veda, knowledge).

Its origin is traced back to the Vedic times about 5000 BC. Ayurveda is a part of the Atharva Veda which solely deals with medicine.

Atharva Veda includes eight divisions of Ayurveda:

1. Kayachikitsa (Internal Medicine)
2. Salakya Tantra (Surgery of Head & neck, Ophthalmology and Otolaryngology).
3. Shalya Tantra (Surgery)
4. Agada Tantra (Toxicology)
5. Bhuta Vidya (Psychiatry)
6. Kaumarabhrity (Pediatric)
7. Rasayana (Anti-aging or Gerontology or Science of Rejuvenation) and
8. Vajkarana (The Science of Fertility)

The Vedic Sages took passages from Atharva Veda and created separate books dealing exclusively with Ayurveda.

Atreya Samhita is the oldest medical book in the world. Atreya was the son of Rishi Atri.

Atri was the son of god Brahma and one of the seven immortal Rishis in Vedic literature.

Rishi Atri was Acharya (Teacher) of Ayurveda.

The Vedic Brahmanas were priests who performed religious rites and ceremonies.

They were also considered as *Vaidyas* (Physicians of Ayurveda).

These sage physicians were the surgeons in the ancient days.

These deeply devoted holy physicians considered health to be an important part of spiritual life.

It is believed that the *Vaidyas* received their training of Ayurveda during meditation which were later transcribed into book form.

Beginning of Medicine and Surgery in India is thought as the gifts from god Indra to Sages Bharadwaja, the patron saint of medicine and Dhanvantari, the patron saint of Surgery.

These two main schools made Ayurveda a more scientifically verifiable medical system (around 1500 BC). These two scholar passed their knowledge to two worthy men Atreya and Susruta. Both Atreya and Susruta practised around 600 BC, nearly 150 years before Hippocrates. Maharshi Atreya is acknowledged as the first great Indian Physician and Teacher. He lived in the ancient University Taxilla about 20 miles west of modern Rawalpindi. He learnt Ayurveda from Rishi Bharadwaja.

Bharadwaja Ashrama still exists in Prayag (in the modern state of Uttar Pradesh). Atreya revolutionized the medical system of Ayurveda into the system we have today. He held formal teachings with his students and established Code of Medical Ethics in India (150 years before Hippocratic oath).

- Agnivesa Samhita (800 BC – 400 AD):

- Agnivesa, one of the six disciples of Atreya, who recorded the teachings of his preceptor Atreya.

- Charaka re-edited Agnivesa Samhita as Charaka Samhita in the second century (200 AD).

- Galen was his contemporary in the West (130–210 AD).

- Charaka Samhiṭa describes Anatomy and Physiology.

- There are eight chapters dealing with Pathology (*Nidanasthanam*).

- Charaka Samhita deals with the symptoms, signs, diagnosis and treatment of diseases of the heart, chest, abdomen, genital organs and extremities.

Charaka mentions two cases of disease:

1. *Internal* - Loss of faith in Devine which leads to suffering in spiritual, mental and physical disease.
2. *External* - varies with time of the day, seasons, diet and life-style.

His profound medical knowledge was evident from his instructions on building hospitals with maintenance of hygienic atmosphere for patients.

Dhanvantri resigned his Royal status as 'Prince of Kasi' (Varanasi) and retired into the forest where he dictated his Ayurveda to Susruta of Benaras. He described human anatomy in details in his treatise "Susruta Samhita".

Susruta was the first surgeon to perform rhinoplasty and ear lobe construction.

Surgeons of that time had plenty of opportunity to construct the nose.

Besides those who lost their nose in the battle, cutting the nose by the irritant 'Rajas' was the common practice.

Official punishment for adultery was to cut the nose of the culprits.

The early Indians set fractures, performed amputations, excised tumors, repaired hernia and did couching for cataract.

They used over 121 different steel instruments to drain fluids, to remove kidney stones, to sew up wounds and to perform plastic surgery. Some of the instruments used in those days were very much like those of today such as scissors, saws, needle, forceps etc.

In Susruta Samhita transmission of malaria was incriminated to a biting insect, probably mosquito. This shows that they were not only well versed in Medicine and surgery but also in the prevention of disease.

They were also conversant with operative midwifery.

Original Susruta Samhita was further revised by Nagarjuna (4th century BC), the great Buddhist Teacher.

The great Greek teacher Hippocrates (460-377 BC) preceded Nagarjuna near about the time of Socrates (469-399 BC).

Susruta Samhita was re-edited by Chakrapani in the 11th Century.

Ancient history of Pathology in India- Nidanasthanam.

Of the six divisions of Susruta Samhita, second division consists of sixteen chapters devoted to Pathology, mainly of surgical diseases.

Nidana developed greatly in the 7th century and was established by Madhava Kara of Bengal.

His Nidana as well as Charaka and Susruta Samhita were translated in Arabic by the order of Haroon Al-Rashid (786-806 AD) the Khalifa of Baghdad.

According to Wilson, it is likely that it might have been translated from the translation of the book in Persian language. Postmortem : In *Arthasastra of Kautilya* (other name of Chanakya, the greatest politician of the time), there is a mention of postmortem. *Ashumrita parikshagara* (examination of men who recently died).

These reports of inquest were also necessary in higher courts of law (*Kontaka Sodhana*) during the reign of the Great Emperor Chandragupta.

The dead bodies in cases of homicide, suicide or those who died of accidents, were kept in an examination room, which was set apart for the purpose and the cause of death had to be reported after post-mortem examination to higher authorities.

To prevent decomposition dead bodies were preserved by immersion in oil.

The Golden Age of Indian Medicine was between 800 BC to 600 AD.

Learned men from different countries such as China, Tibet, Afghanistan, the Greeks, Romans, Egyptians, Persians came to the Indian Ayurvedic Schools to learn about this World Medicine.

Ayurvedic texts were translated into Arabic by the physicians like Avicenna and Razi Sempion.

Both of them quoted Indian Ayurvedic texts and established Islamic medicine "Unani System".

This Indian Ayurvedic System became popular in Europe and helped to form the foundation of the European tradition of medicine.

Ayurveda grew tremendously during Buddhist Kings like King Ashoka (226 BC), who patronized Ayurveda as State Medicine and established Schools of Medicine and Hospitals.

Charaka (200 AD),the most popular name in Ayurveda medicine was the Court Physician to the Buddhist king Kaniska during Buddhist time.

Due to the doctrine of "*Ahinsa*" (non-violence) Indian Surgery suffered a setback.

With the advent of Muslims in India, Indian Medicine eroded due to the lack of State help and support by the rulers.

Unani system of medicine was introduced into India by the Muslim rulers.

By the 13th Century Unani system of medicine was firmly established mainly in Delhi, Aligarh, Lucknow and Hyderabad.

During Mughal period and subsequent years Ayurveda declined due to the lack of state support.

With the advent of the British in the 18th Century Ayurveda system was revived in India along with Western system of Medicine.

Chinese medicine claims to be the world's first organised body of medical knowledge dating back to 2700 BC. The Chinese system of so-called bare foot doctors, and acupuncture anaesthesia have attracted world-wide attention.

Like prehistoric medicine in India, Egyptian medicine also dates from 2000 BC.

Edwin Smith's papyrus of 1600 BC described fractures, dislocation, infection of wounds, tumors etc.

The best known medical manuscript is the Ebers papyrus(1500 BC) found with the Mummy on the bank of the Nile.

It mentions coryza, disease of the bones and joints, tumors, disease of the gastrointestinal tract, female genitalia, eye, etc.

Egyptians had no foundation of anatomical knowledge.

Alexandria in Egypt had their medical schools in temples of their God of Medicine Imhotep.

All doctors were paid by the State.

Homer while speaking of the doctors of the ancient world, considered the Egyptians to be the best of all.

Egyptian medicine dominated for about 2500 years when it was replaced by the Greek medicine.

The Greek invaded Asia minor and were influenced by the medical knowledge of Mesopotamia and Egypt.

Early leader in Greek medicine, Asculapius (2000 BC) was the Greek god of medicine.

The staff of Asculapius with a single serpent coiled around it represents the Medical Profession.

Modern winged staff with twin snakes around a single staff is the "wand of Hermes" (Greek messenger god or Roman god Mercury).

Greatest Greek physician Hippocrates (460-370 BC) set a high standard of moral behaviour for medical man.

When the pupil of Hippocrates became doctors they had to swear an oath:

> 'Thou would help the sick according to their ability and judgement, never give poisons, not tell other people what their patients had told them and keep both themselves and their profession pure'.

This 'Oath of Hippocrates' still goes by 'International Oath'.

It sets a high moral standard for the medical profession and demand absolute integrity of doctors.

The Greek civilization fell into decay and was succeeded by the Roman civilization by the 1st century BC.

The Roman borrowed their medicine from the Greeks.

Celsus (25 BC to 50 AD) has given us the cardinal signs of inflammation.

Galen (13 to 105 AD) was the pioneer of Experimental Medicine.

He observed that the disease was due to:

- Predisposing factors
- Exciting factors and
- Environmental factors.

This is the true modern idea. His writings were accepted as standard text books in medicine for centuries after his death.

With the fall of Roman Empire, Roman school of medicine disappeared.

The practice of medicine reverted back to primitive medicine dominated by superstition and dogma.

This period (500 to 1500 AD.) is called the 'Dark Age of Medicine'. During this period Arabs stole a march over the rest of the civilization.

Graeco-Roman Medical literature was translated into Arabic & they developed their own system of medicine known as 'Unani System of Medicine'.

They founded medical schools and hospitals in Baghdad, Damascus, Cairo and other Muslim capitals.

'The Golden Age of Arabian Medicine' was between 800 to 1300 AD.

Medical historians admit that there was interchange of thought and experience between Hindu, Arab, Persian, Greek and Jewish scholars.

Gradual spread of Christianity led to the establishment of religious institutions known as "Monasteries".(Headed by religious leaders known as monks, saints and abbotts). These Monasteries also rendered active medical and nursing care to the sick.

As human knowledge advanced, medicine was revived by Paracelsus (1490-1541),who removed superstition and dogma in medicine.

Andreas Vesalius (1514-1564) did a lot of dissections on the human body and demonstrated some of Galen's errors.

Till the eighteenth century the teaching and practice of medicine in India was done according to the Ayurvedic or ancient Vedic Hindu system and the Unani or Arabic system based on the Egyptian and Greecian schools and brought to India by the Greek and Muslim rulers.

The wisdom and seniority of the great teachers Charaka and Susruta compared to the pioneer western physicians like Hippocrates and other famous Greek physicians were accepted universally not only in basic medical sciences, therapeutics and surgery but also in laying down the ethical code for practice of medicine and nursing.

In the early 19th century, the British Government of India could not entrust the health care of their own people in the hands of Ayurveda and Unani practitioners and they had to bring medical men from Europe.

The British Surgeons trained a few Indians the elementary principles of diagnosis and treatment of disease and appointed them as Native Doctors to help them as compounders and dressers.

They received no systematic education but had to pass through tests before being entitled to higher pay and responsibilities.

The services of these dedicated men were soon appreciated by the British Surgeons and in 19th May 1822, the Medical Board of the British Surgeons wrote to the then Secretary to the

Government of India for a more systematic education for the Native doctors which was formally approved on 24th May 1882.

With a Government Order dated 21st June, 1822, the first Medical School in British India was established.

The School opened in October, 1824 at Calcutta Sanskrit College with Dr. James Jamieson as the first Superintendent.

The students also learnt side by side the great works of Charaka and Susruta as well as those of Avicenna and other physicians of the Arabic School.

The Charaka Samhita lays down an elaborate code regarding the lays down an elaborate code regarding the training, duties, privilege and social status of physicians. It can be considered as the origin of medical ethics. Students were selected for training on fixed criteria, and instructions were given free. The 'Charaka Samhita' gives a detailed description of various poisons, symptoms, signs and treatments of poisoning.

Susruta wrote his Samhita, the most authentic text on the practice of Ayurvedic surgery around the sixth century BC Susruta is, also, renowned as the father of surgery. In Samhita chapters pertaining to forensic medicine were so carefully written that they are in no way inferior to modern knowledge on the subject. It also contains a separate chapter on toxicology. The poisons were classified into:

1. Plant products
2. Animal products, and
3. Artificial.

Not only were the symptoms signs and treatment of poisoning described in detail, but also modes of administration of poisons, character of the poisoner and examination of suspected poisonous materials. A poisoner could be known from his behaviour and movements – he will not answer to questions, will keep silent, talk irrelevantly and so on. Poisons were administered through food and drinks; tooth stick; oils and materials for message; medicaments; water for bathing; articles of clothing; snuffs; smokes and surmas. Emetics and their use are mentioned. The duty of the physician was to save the king from any poisoning or *Visha Kanya-* the poisonous damsel. Qualities, responsibilities and duties of physicians were defined. Shusruta is unique on chapters on injuries, pregnancy and delivery. Types of weapons and foreign bodies, the signs and symptoms they manifest in the body has also been described. Wounds and fracture of bones have been classified. Principles of cohabitation, signs in a woman fit for conception after periods; signs immediately after impregnation and signs of pregnancy have been mentioned. Among these are darkening of areola and nipple, dropping of eyelids, vomiting without any cause, salivation, and tiredness over the body. Delivery, abortions and foetal development at various months of pregnancy has been very accurately described.

In Muslim period in India the criminal laws were well developed and became a landmark. At that period 'Quasi-I-Mumalik' was in charge of civil and criminal litigations. His function was to find out facts and apply the law. There were so many defects in the Muslim criminal law which were detected by the British and were even abolished.

The first recorded medico-legal autopsy was performed in India by Dr. Edward Bulkley on the afternoon of 28 August 1693.

Deep-rooted national prejudice was the great hurdle to the study of Anatomy or dissection. Professor Goodeve started demonstration of the parts of human body using sheep's brain, goat's liver and human skeletons. Two skeletons were purchased through Messrs.

On 10th January 1836 Pandit Madhusudan Gupta, accompanied by four young students followed Professor Goodeve to an outhouse of the Medical College building & began to dissect a dead body with his own hands. This day will ever be marked in the Annals of Western Medicine in India when Indians rose superior to all prejudice and boldly flung open the gates of modern scientific medicine to fellow countrymen.

In less than 2 years there was rapid advancement in the art of dissection. In 1848, Professor Goodeve remarked in his introductory lecture that his pupils have dissected more than 500 bodies.

Though the Medical College was established in 1835, Medical Jurisprudence was not in the curriculum.

In 1845, the system was re-modelled and Dr. F.J Mouat was entrusted to teach Medical Jurisprudence.

In 1850, an independent chair was created and Dr. C.T.O. Woodford was the first Professor (1850-1860).

During this period, Dr. Norman Chevers wrote a valuable treatise on the subject which became the college text book.

Professor S.C. Mackenzie (1879-1894) did original work on "Changes on dead bodies" in and around Calcutta, which is accepted as the guideline in establishing the time since death in Courts of Law.

The Science of Dactylography was started in Bengal and the Finger Print Bureau was started in Calcutta in 1897 with the active help of Professors of Medical Jurisprudence.

In 1892, the Central Medical Council of Great Britain recognized the medical degrees of Calcutta University.

In 1906, L.M.S. course was abolished and from 1907 M.B. degree course was introduced. Henceforth, Medical Jurisprudence was included in the course.

The Professor of Medical Jurisprudence was also the Police Surgeon of Calcutta.

In 1938, the post of the Police Surgeon was created and the Professor of Medical Jurisprudence was relieved of the duties of the Police Surgeon.

The most outstanding contribution of India to legal medicine during burnish period is modern dactylography. It was Sir William Herschel of the Indian Civil Services, who first used this method of identification in 1858. Based on Herschel's theory. Sir Francis Galton of England devised the systemic study and methods of using fingerprints for personal identification in 1892.

The British government altered this law from time to time till 1862 when the Indian penal Code came into existence. Four law Commissioners of whom Lard Macaulay was the chief, prepared the draft Penal Code and submitted to the Governor-General in Counsel on 14th October 1837. On 26th April 1845, it was sent to a Commission of two gentlemen to be revised in the light of English Law, which was then intended to modify and for which a similar Commission had been then sitting in English. This Commission submitted two reports, dated 5th Nov 1846 and 24th June 1847. The Bill as revised was pigeon hold for twelve or more years and was passed into law only on 6th October 1860. The code as enacted was different from the Bill prepared by the law Commissioner who had recommended only 488 while the code as enacted contained 511 sections.

The Indian Medical Council was established in 1933. The police system of crime investigation was introduced in India in 1861 and the coroners systems in 1871 in the presidency towns of Bombay and Calcutta.

In the late 20th century, in many medical disciplines doctors have benefited from the revolutionary development of digital computers and their automated information management and analytical capabilities.

Medical science has evolved over many centuries from the pre-Vedic era to the present time.

Recently the teaching of forensic medicine has improved with the establishment and expansion of the academic departments of forensic medicine and toxicology: in most of the medical colleges. Postgraduate courses in forensic medicine an available in several universities.

By using newer methods of computer and information sciences, anatomists, histopathologists and radiologists have made outstanding contributions to science, medicine, and education.

Mastering computer sciences and informatics methods is essential for the present generation of doctors, who will shape the future in research, clinical knowledge, and teaching.

General Aspects of Medical Jurisprudence:

1. Persons authorized to perform autopsies: a) health officers, b) medical officers of law enforcement agencies, and c) members of the medical staff of accredited hospitals.
2. Autopsies shall be performed in the following cases: a) whenever required by special laws, b) upon order of a competent court, a mayor and a provincial or city fiscal, c) upon written request of police authorities, d) whenever the Solicitor General, provincial or city fiscal deem it necessary to disinter and take possession of the remains for examination to determine the cause of death, and e) whenever the nearest kin shall request in writing the authorities concerned to ascertain the cause and nature of death.

Definition of Medical Evidence

It is species of proof, or probative matter, legally presented at the trial of an issue by the act of the parties, and through the medium of witnesses, records, documents, concrete objects, etc. for the purpose of inducing belief in the minds of the court as their contention. If the means employed to prove a fact is medical in nature then it becomes medical evidence.

Types of Medical Evidence

Hereunder are the types of medical evidences:

1. Testimonial Evidence

A physician may be commended to appear before a court to give his testimony. While in the witness stand, he is obliged to answer questions propounded by counsel and presiding officer of the court. His testimony must be given orally and under oath or affirmation.

2. Physical Evidence

These are articles and materials which are found in connection with the investigation and which aid in establishing the identity of the perpetrator or the circumstances under which the crime was committed, or in general assist in the prosecution of a criminal.

3. Autoptic or Real Evidence

This is evidence made known or addressed to the sense of the court. It is not limited to that which is known through the sense of vision but is extended to what the sense of hearing, smell and touch is perceived.

4. Documentary Evidence

A document is an instrument on which is recorded by means of letters, figures, or marks intended to be used for the purpose of recording that matter which may be evidentially used. The term applies to writings, to words printed, lithographed or photographed; to seals, plates or stones on which inscriptions are cut or engraved; to photographs and pictures to maps or plans.

5. Experimental Evidence

A medical witness may be allowed by the court to confirm his allegation or as a corroborated proof to an opinion he previously stated.

Preservation of Medical Evidence

The physical evidences recovered during medico-legal investigation must be preserved to maintained their value when presented as exhibits in court. Most medical evidences are easily destroyed or physically or chemically altered unless appropriate preservation procedure is applied. This problem is further compounded by the long space of the time the evidence was recovered and its presentation in court.

From its recovery and from becoming a part of the investigation report, a preliminary investigation will be made by the prosecuting fiscal to prove that there is a *prima facie* evidence to warrant the filing of information of the case in court. While in court, preferential trials of other cases, raisings of prejudicial issues to higher courts, etc., preservation of evidence is indeed vital in medico-legal investigation.

Methods of Preserving Medical Evidence

The following are some of the most common methods of preserving medical evidence:

1. Description

This is putting into words the person or thing to be preserved. Describing a thing requires keen observation and a good power of attention, perception, intelligence and experience. It must cause a vivid impression on the mind of the reader, a true picture of the thing described.

2. Photography

Photography is considered to be the most practical, useful and reliable means of preservation. In colored photographs, variations may occur in the choice of the kind of film and printing paper.

3. Sketching

If no scientific apparatus to preserve evidence is available, a rough drawing of the scene or object to be preserve is done. It must be simple, identifying significant items and with exact measurements.

4. Mannequin Method

It is a miniature model of a scene or of a human body indicating marks of the various aspects of the things to be preserved. An anatomical model or statuette may be used and injuries are indicated with their appropriate legends.

5. Preservation in the Mind of Witness

A person who perceives something relevant for proper adjudication of a case may be a witness in court if he has the power to transmit to others what he perceived. He would just have to make a recital of his collection.

6. Special Methods

Special way of treating certain types of evidence may be necessary. Preservation may be essential for the time it is recovered to make the condition unchanged up to the period it reaches the criminal laboratory for appropriate examination. Preservation may be needed for the remaining portion of the evidence submitted for court verification.

Weight and Sufficiency of Medical Evidence

In civil cases, the party having the burden of proof must established is case by a preponderance of evidence. In determining where the preponderance or superior weight of evidence on the issues involved lies, the court may consider all the facts and circumstances of the case, the witnesses' manner of testifying, their intelligence, their means and opportunity of knowing the facts to which they are testifying, the nature of the facts to which they testify, the probability and improbability of their testimony, their interest or want of interest, and also their personal credibility so far as the same may legitimately appear upon the trial.

The court may also consider the number of witnesses, though the preponderance is not necessarily with the greatest number. From the foregoing provision of the Rules of Court, the following factors must be considered which party's evidence preponderance: 1. all the facts and circumstances of the case, 2. the witnesses manner of testifying, their intelligence, their means and opportunities of knowing the facts to which they are testifying, 3. the nature of the facts to which the witnesses testify, 4. the probability and improbability of the witnesses; testimony, 5. the interest or want of interest of the witnesses, 6. credibility of the witness so far as the same may legitimately appear upon the trial, and 7. the number of witnesses presented, although preponderance is not necessarily with the greatest number.

In a criminal case, the defendant is entitled to an acquittal, unless his guilt is shown beyond reasonable doubt. Proof beyond reasonable doubt does not mean such a degree of proof as, excluding possibility of error, produces absolute certainty. Moral certainty only is required, or that degree of proof which produces conviction in an unprejudiced mind. It is presumed that a person is innocent of crime until the contrary is proven beyond reasonable doubt.

The doubt, the benefit of which an accused is entitled in a criminal case, is a reasonable doubt, and not a whimsical or fanciful doubt, based on imagined and wholly improbable possibilities and unsupported by evidence. In this, sufficiency-of-evidence refers to principle that helps determining the accusation. Sufficiency of medical evidence in crimes against person is a standard in reviewing a criminal conviction. When a case involves new criminal charges that were not tested at the preliminary hearing, the appropriate test for review of the new charge requires the test for the sufficiency of medical test.

2
Aspects of Identification

Medical Jurisprudence literally evolves on the corpus delicti. It begins with the aspects of identification and proceeds through history, physical examination, and even laboratory tests. The key goal is to provide objective evidence of cause, timing, and manner of death in the administration of justice.

Above all, the law enforcement agencies during investigation want to know whether the bones collected at the crime scene were human or animal. Usually it is a fact of establishing corpus delicti. They have to keep in mind that all bones, especially fragmentary, look alike to untrained observers.

Definition of Identification of Person

Identification of person are a task of identifying a particular person out of a group of people based on physiology cues such as speech, facial images, finger- prints and iris, etc. based on facial image, the identification of person is also called face identification. Either category has been extensively addressed, and is traditionally formulated as a pattern recognition problem in some feature vector space, tackled by statistical classification and machine learning algorithms.

Bases of Person's Identification

The bases of person's identification may be classified as:

1. Those which laymen used to prove identity : no special training or skill is required of the identifier and no instrument or procedure is demanded.

2. Those which are based on scientific knowledge; identification is made by trained men, well-seasoned by experience and observation, and primarily based on comparison of exclusion.

Extrinsic Factors in Identification

Hereunder are some extrinsic factors in identification of individual persons are as follows:

1. *Ornamentation:* rings, bracelet, necklace, hairpin, earrings, lapel pin, etc., and identification by close friends and relatives.
2. *Personal belongings:* letters, wallet, driver's licenses, residence certificate, personal cards, etc., and identification records on file at the police station, immigration bureau, hospitals, etc.
3. *Wearing apparel:* tailor marks, laundry mark, printed name of owner, size, style, and texture, footwear, socks, more particularly with embroidered lettering or symbols.
4. *Foreign bodies:* dust in clothing, cerumen in the ears, nail scraping may show occupation or profession, place of residence or work, habit, etc.
5. *Identification photographs or thru superimposed photography:* a special method of determining the facial configuration of a person to whom the skull belongs.

Light as a Factor in Identification:

The following are factors to be considered in the identification through:

1. *Flash of Lighting*

The flash of lighting produces sufficient light for the identification of an individual provided that person's eye is focused towards the individual he wishes to identity during the flash.

2. *Artificial Light*

In case of artificial light, the identity is relative to the kind and intensity of the light. Experiments may be made for every particular artificial light concerned.

3. Flash of Firearm

Although by experiment, letters of two inches high can be read with the aid of the flash of a caliber .22 firearms at a distance of two feet it is hardly possible for a witness to see the assailant in case of a hold-up that is hidden.

4. Broad Daylight

A person can hardly recognized another person at a distance farther than one hundred yards if the person has never been seen before, but persons who are almost strangers may be recognized at a distance of twenty-five yards.

5. Clearest Moonlight or Starlight

Various experiments conducted have shown that the best known person cannot be recognized by the clearest moon light at a distance than sixteen to seventeen yards and by starlight any further than ten to thirteen yards.

Dental Identification

The role of the teeth in human identification is important for the following reasons:

1. The possibility of two persons to have the same dentition is quite remote. This is due to the fact that human, more particularly the adults has thirty-two teeth and each tooth gas five surfaces.
2. Some of the teeth may be missing, carious, with filling materials, and with abnormality in shape and other peculiarities. This will lead to several combination with almost infinite in number of the dental characteristics of individual person.
3. The enamel of the teeth is the hardest substance of the human body. It may outlast all other tissues during putrefaction or physical destruction.
4. The more recent the ante-mortem records of the persons to be identified the more reliable is the comparative or exclusionary mode of identification that can be done.

5. After death, the greater the degree of tissue destruction, the grater is the importance of dental characteristics as a means of positive identification.
6. The more recent the ante-mortem records of the persons to be identified the more reliable is the comparative or exclusionary mode of identification that can be done.

In order to make an accurate dental record available for purposes of comparison with that of the person to be identified, practitioners may seek reference to dentistry or keep records of their patients.

Identification of Skeleton

Occasionally, before a physician is called to examine a dead body, the soft tissues have already disappeared and only the skeletal system remains. In this particular case, the study of bones must be resorted. In the examination of bones, the following points can be determined approximately:

1. Whether the remains are of human origin or not. The shape, size and general nature of the remains and especially that of the head must be studied. The oval or round shape of the skull and the less prominent lower jaw and nasal bone are suggestive of human remains.

   A complete layout of the whole bones found and placing each of them on their corresponding places in the human body will be helpful. The presence of dental fixtures, rings on the fingers, earrings in the case of women, hair and other wearing apparels, together with the remains are strong presumption of human remains.

2. Whether the remains belong to one person or not. A complete layout of the bones on a table in their exact location in the human body is necessary. Any plurality or excess of the bones after a complete lay-out denotes that the remains belong to more than one person. However, congenital deformities as supplementary fingers and toes must be forgotten. The un-equality in sizes, especially of the limbs may be ante-mortem.

3. Determination of height, sex, race, and age. Several formulate using different constants have been forwarded in the approximation of the height of a person by measuring the long bones of the body. In determining the sex skeleton, the following bones must be studied, i.e., pelvis, skull, sternus, femur, and humerus.

It is becoming more difficult to determine the race because of the amalgamation of races. For practical consideration there is hardly no races that is absolutely pure. The following points may be used in determining the race in the remains of a person, i.e., extrinsic factors such as, color of the skin, facial features, nature of the hair, and mode of dressing; indices such as skull, pelvis, and extremities such as crural index, intermembral index, and humero-femoral index.

Aside from the size of the bones and through the conduct of dental examination, the height, age, sex, race of the person to whom the skeleton belongs may be determined by: appearance of the ossification centers, union of bones and epihyses, dental identification, and obliteration of cranial structures.

4. Determination of the duration of internment. The period from the time of death up to the time of examination may be determined by the nature and presence of the soft tissues and the degree or erosion of the bones, ordinarily, all the soft tissues in a grace disappear within a year after internment.
5. Ante-mortem or post-mortem bone injuries. Individual bones must be examined to detail the possible fractures. Importance must be laid on whether these injuries in the bones occurred during life or in the process of exhumation. Note the presence of vital reaction, principally the signs of repairs.

Determination of Sex

Below are some important factors to be considered in the determination of:

1. Legal Importance of Sex Determination

a. As an aid in identification, the habit, social life, manner of dressing, physical features and inclination are generally dependent on the sex. These points are useful in identification.

b. To determine whether an individual can exercise certain obligations vested by law to one sex only. For example, under the National defense Act in several countries, compulsory military service or training refers only to males, twenty years of age or above.

c. Marriage or the union of any male or female at the age of respectively, twenty one and eighteen, may contract marriage. The Hindu Marriage Act of 1955 is applicable to Hindus, Jains, Sikhs and Buddhists. The Hindu Marriage Act provides for the conditions of a marriage where under the bridegroom should be the age of 21 years and bride of 18 years, they both should not be within the degree of prohibited relationship.

However, there were many disparities among the Child Marriage (Restraint) Act, the Hindu Marriage Act, The Indian Christian Marriage Act, 1872, The Shariat and Muslim Personal Law, The Special Marriage Act, 1954, explanation to Section 375 of the Indian Penal Code, the Indian Divorce Act, the Child Labour (Regulation) Act and the Juvenile Justice (Care and Protection of Children) Act, 2000 on the minimum age for marriage of girls.

d. Rights granted by law are different in different sexes.

e. There are certain crimes wherein a specific sex can only be the offender or victim. There are certain cases that are only applicable to women, such as a rape, prostitution, adultery, and violence against women and children.

2. Test to Determine the Sex

a. Social Test: Difference in the social role of the sexes used to be clearly marked but now they are less than they used to be. Dress, hairstyle, general bodily shape provides an immediate and accurate answer to the vast majority of cases.

b. Gonadal Test: Presence of testes in male and ovary in female – this will involve exploration of the abdomen and in some cases a histological examination of the gonad to see whether its microscopic structure is characteristically ovarian or testicular.

c. *Chromosomal Test:* It is noticed that there was a difference between cell derived from men and women suitably stained and examined under the microscope. The nucleus of the cells is a densely staining area in the cell itself and that there was a small part of nucleus which stained deeply that the rest in women's cells but not cell from men. It is observed in the while cells from the blood cells obtained by scrapping the mucous membrane of the mouth. this is Barr bodies.

3. Evidence of Sex

a. Presumptive Evidence, i.e., general features and contour of the face; presence or absence of hair is some parts of the body; length of scalp hair. Generally, the female has long hair in the scalp than that of the male; clothes and other wearing apparel, but not in a transvestite; figure females have prominent pelvis, while those of the males are slender; habit or inclination, pseudo-hermaphrodites are person who have the gonadad tissue of one sex and the behavior of the opposite sex; and voice and manner of speech.

b. Highly probable evidences of sex, i.e., possession of vagina, uterus, and accessories in female, and penis in male; presence of developed and large breasts in female; and muscular development distribution of fat in the body.

c. Conclusive evidence, i.e., presence of ovary in females and testis in males.

d. Evidence of sex in mutilated or decomposed body, i.e., general physical and muscular development; hairline of the scalp, face, chest, pubes, and other parts of the body; prominence of the Adam's apple; amount of subcutaneous fat in specific part of the body; presence of linea albicantes, enlarge nipple, cutex in fingernails and lipsticks or coloring materials; and presence of prostate gland in male or uterus and ovary in female. If in doubt, a microscopic examination must be made on the suspicious ovarian or testicular tissue.

4. Problem in Sex Determination

Sex determination may be possible and can scientifically be distinguished on account of the biological structure differences;

however, in the following instances there will be no way to determine the sex:

a. *Gonadal Agenesis:* Sex organs, testes or ovaries, have never developed.

b. *True Hermaphrodism:* A state of bi-sexuality—the gonads of both sexes were present which may be separated or combined as ovotestis.

Determination of Age

For age determination, the following points have to take into considerations, as follows:

1. *Legal Importance of Determination of Age*

a. Determination of criminal liability. Circumstances which exempt from criminal liability. The following are exempted from criminal liability, i.e., a person under nine years of age; and a person over nine years of age and under fifteen, unless he has acted with discernment, especially for atrocities against women, in which case, such minor, shall be proceeded against in accordance with provision of the Juvenile Justice (Care and Protection of Children) Act, 2015.

b. As an aid in identification. Mention of the age of the wanted or missing person will create an impression of the physical characteristics, social life, and psychic and mental behavior of that person. Although it may only be presumptive, it may be useful in identification.

c. Determination of the exercise civil rights. Majority commences upon the attainment of the age of twenty-one (21) years. The person who had reached majority is qualified for all act of civil life, save the exceptional established by the Civil Code in special cases.

d. As a requisite to certain crimes. This involves crimes of rape, infanticide, seductions, and consented abduction, violence against women, and in instances of child abuse and exploitation.

2. Determination of the Age of the Fetus

a. Application of the Hess's of Haases Rule. For foetus of less 25 cm. long, get the square root of the length in centimeter and the result is the age of the foetus in month. For foetus 25 cm. or more, divide the length of the foetus by 5, and the results is the age in month.

b. Examination of the product of conception. This can be done by determining the months of conception, and the nature of the product of conception.

3. Age Determination During Infancy

a. Age based on height of weight. The estimation of the age utilizing the weight and/or the height is not quite useful inasmuch as there is a difference in the rapidity of growth not only in children of different sex, but also children of the same sex.

b. Physical characteristics of infant. The skin of a newly born are covered with vernix caeosa and red, meconium present in the rectum, lanugo hair almost disappeared, and limbs and body plumps.

c. Age determination in childhood and adulthood are as follows: 1) age based on the eruption of teeth, 2) appearance of ossification centers, 3) union of epiphysis with shaft of bones, and 4) obliteration of cranial structure.

Role of Medico Legal Officer in Establishing Identity

Establishing the identity of a person may seem like an easy task; the person, or their friends or family, can simply be asked their name. In medico-legal cases, there are often reasons why people are either unable to give accurate answers. In cases of death, a body may also be too disfigured due to trauma to allow for easy identification.

Though sometimes difficult, identification remains a necessary task. Living individuals for whom identification is required may include wanted criminals attempting victims, or persons who require identity confirmation. Deceased individuals requiring identification may include burned bodies, decomposed or skeletal remains, and individuals who sustained significant facial trauma that precludes visual identification.

Just as identification of a living individual allows for contacting of next of kin if necessary, or processing their medical/legal needs, identification of a deceased person serves many purposes. Family can be contacted, allowing for the grieving process to begin and permitting arrangements for disposition of the body. Death investigation is greatly enhanced by knowing the identity of the person.

3

Medico-legal Aspects of Death

The medico-legal aspects of death are responsible for conducting death investigations and certifying the cause and manner of unnatural and unexplained deaths. Unnatural and unexplained deaths include homicides, suicides, unintentional injuries, drug-related deaths, and other deaths that are sudden or unexpected.

Overview of Medico Legal Aspect of Death

Death investigations carry broad societal importance for criminal justice and public health. Death investigations provide evidence to convict the guilty and protect the innocent, whether they are accused of murder, child maltreatment, neglect, or other crimes. Death investigations are critical for many aspects, most often in injury prevention and control, and also in suicide, violence, etc.

Death investigations are emerging as critically important in evaluating the quality of health care and the nation's response to bio-terrorism. The term medico- legal aspects of death are something of a misnomer. It is an umbrella term for a patchwork of highly varied state and local systems for investigating deaths. Death investigations are carried out by the medical legal examiners.

The role of the medico-legal aspect of death is to decide the scope and course of a death investigation, which includes, i.e., examining the body, determining whether to perform an autopsy, and ordering x-ray, toxicology, or other laboratory tests. Medical examiners are physicians, pathologists, or forensic pathologists with jurisdiction over a particular place. They bring medical expertise to the evaluation of the medical history and physical examination of the deceased.

Definition of Death

Death is the termination of life. It is the complete cessation of all the vital functions without possibility of resuscitation. It is an irreversible of the properties of the living matter. Dying is a continuing process while death is an event that takes place at a precise time. The ascertainment of death is a clinical and not a legal problem.

Criteria in the Determination of Death

Enumerated and discussed hereunder are some of the criteria used by the medico legal examiners in the determination of death:

1. *Brain Death*

Death occurs when there is irreversible coma, absence of electrical brain activity and complete cessation of all the vital functions without possibility of resuscitation.

2. *Cardio-Respiratory Death*

Death occurs when there is a continuous and persistent cessation of heart action and respiration. Cardio-respiratory death is a condition in which the physician and the members of the family pronounced a person to be death based on the common sense and intuition.

3. *Others*

Some countries or states provide both brain and cardio-respiratory bases in an alternative or electric way in the determination of death. Phenomena which commonly bring about death include old age, predation, malnutrition, disease, suicide, murder and accidents or trauma resulting in terminal injury.

Kinds of Death

In addition to the criteria used in the determination of death, hereunder are kinds of death:

1. *Somatic Death or Clinical Death*

This is the state of the body in which there is complete, persistent and continuous cessation of the vital functions of the brain, heart and lungs that maintain life and health. It occurs the moment the physician or other members of the family declare a person has expired, and some of the early signs of death are present. It is hardly possible to determine the exact time of death.

Immediately after death the face and lips become pale, the muscles become flaccid, the sphincters are relax, the lower jaw tends to drop, the eyelids remain open, pupils dilated, and the skin losses its elasticity. The body fluid tends to gravitate to the most depended portions of the body, and the body heat gradually assumes the temperature of the surrounding environment.

2. *Molecular or Cellular Death*

After cessation of the vital functions of the body there is still animal life along individual cells. This is evidence by the presence of excitability of muscles and cilliary's movements and other functions of individual cells.

About three to six hours, later, there is death of individual cells. This is known as molecular or cellular death. Its exact occurrence cannot definitely ascertain because its time of appearance is influenced by several factors, i.e., previous state of health, infection, climatic condition, cellular nutrition, etc.

3. *Apparent Death or State of Suspended Animation*

This condition is not really death but merely a transient loss of consciousness or temporary cessation of the vital functions of the body on account of disease, external stimulus or other forms of influence. It may arise especially in hysteria, uremia, catalepsy and electric shock.

It may be induced voluntarily and be able to pass into a state of pulse-less of half an hour. Involuntary suspension is shown stillbirth. A newly born child may remain at the state of suspended animation and may die unless prompt action is taken. A person who has been rescued from drowning may appear dead but life is maintained after continuous resuscitation.

Signs of Death

To guide not only the medical jurist, but the law enforcers of the early indications of death, hereunder are some early signs of death:

1. Cessation of Heart Action and Circulation

There must be an entire and continuous cessation of the heart action and flow of blood in the whole vascular system. A temporary suspension of the heart action is still compatible with life. The length of the time the heart may cease to function and life is still maintained depends upon the oxygenation of blood at the time of the suspension. As a general rule, if there is no heart action for a period of five minutes, death is regarded as certain.

Respiration ceases frequently before the stoppage of the heart contraction and circulation. Usually the auricle of the heart contracts after somatic death for a longer period than the ventricle. And the auricle is the last to stop, hence called -ultimen mariens. In judicial hanging, the heart continues to beat twenty minutes or half an hour after the individual has been executed although its beating is irregular and feeble. In decapitation, heart beating is present for an hour after decapitation has taken place.

2. Cessation of Respiration

Like heart action, cessation of respiration in order to be considered a signs of death must be continuous and persistent. A person can hold his breath for a period not longer than 3 ½ minutes. In case of electrical shock, respiration may cease for sometimes but may be restored by continuous artificial respiration.

The following are the instances of suspension of respiration: 1) in a purely voluntary act, as in divers, swimmers, etc., but it cannot be longer than two minutes, 2) in some peculiar condition of respiration, like Cheyne-Strokes respiration, but the apneic interval cannot be longer than fifteen to twenty seconds, 3) in case of apparent drowning, and 4) newly-born infants may not breathe for a time after birth and may commence only after stimulation or spontaneously later.

3. Cooling of the Body-Rigor Mortis

After death the metabolic process inside the body ceases. No more heat is produced, and the body loses slowly its temperature by evaporation or by conductions to the surrounding atmosphere. The progressive fall of body temperature is one of the most prominent signs of death.

The rate of cooling of the body is not uniform. It is rapid during the first two hours after death and as the temperature of the body gradually approaches the temperature of the surrounding, the rate becomes slower. It is difficult to tell exactly the length of time the body will assume the temperature of the surroundings. Several factors influence the rate of fall of body temperature.

The fall of temperature may occur before death in the following conditions, i.e., cancer, pthisis, and collapse. The fall of temperature of 15 to 20 degrees Fahrenheit are considered as a certain sign of death. Post-mortem caloricity is the rise of temperature of the body after death due to rapid and early putrefactive changes or some internal changes. It is usually observed in the first two hours after death.

Estimates of the Cooling of the Body

a. When the body temperature is normal at the time of death, the average rate of fall of the temperature during the first two hours is one-half of the difference of the body temperature and that of the air.

During the next hours, the temperature fall is one-half of the previous rates, and during the succeeding two hours, it is one-half of the last mentioned rates. As a general rule the body attains the temperature of the surrounding environment from 12 to 15 hours after death in tropical countries.

b. Normal body temperature is 98.6 degrees Fahrenheit. After death, the body loses or gains heat progressively until it equilibrates with that of the surrounding medium. Since corpse temperature can be easily and quickly obtained, the search for a formula that uses this parameter to define the time of death has been sought for years. As early as 1839, English physician John Davey undertook the study of corpse heat loss in London, and as late as 1962, T.K. Marshall and F.E. Hoare attempted to standardize this analysis when they established a computerized mathematical formula known as the Standard Cooling Curve. In the intervening years, and even since Marshall and Hoare, many others have attempted to devise similar schemes. Unfortunately, none of these have proven to be any more accurate than the current formula for heat loss of 1.5 degree per hour.

The formula is:

Hours since death = 98.6 – corpse core temperature/1.5

This approximate rate of heat loss continues until the environmental temperature is attained, after which it remains stable. That sounds simple enough.

Unfortunately, it's not quite that straight forward. The 1.5-degree-per-hour factor varies, depending upon the environment surrounding the body, the size of the corpse, clothing, and other factors. For example, a body in a temperate room will lose heat much more slowly than will one in an icy, flowing stream. And a body in a hot environment, such as an enclosed garage in Phoenix, Arizona, in August, where the ambient temperature could be 125 degrees Fahrenheit or more, will gain heat. The key is that the corpse will lose or gain heat until it reaches equilibrium with its environment.

The coroner's technician who processes the corpse at the scene takes a body temperature, and also measures the temperature of the surrounding medium—air, water, snow, or soil (if the body is buried). Ideally, the body temperature is taken either rectally or by measuring the liver temperature, which may be a more accurate reflection of the true core body temperature. This requires making a small incision in the upper right abdomen and passing the thermometer into the tissue of the liver. This should only be done by a trained individual and under the direction of the medical examiner. Care should be taken not to alter or destroy any existing wounds on the body. Some people have suggested measuring the core temperature by inserting the thermometer into a knife wound or gunshot injury to negate the need to make a new incision. This should never be done because the introduction of any foreign object may contaminate or alter the wound, which can be key evidence in the case. For practical reasons, the rectal temperature is usually taken.

The sooner after death the body is found, the more accurately time of death can be assessed by this method. Once the body reaches ambient temperature, all bets are off. But even if done correctly and soon after death, body temperature determination is subject to several sources of inaccuracy.

One assumption made in the calculations is the initial body temperature. The normal 98.6 degrees Fahrenheit is an average and varies from person to person. Some people have higher normal temperatures than others. Women tend to run higher temperatures than do men. Illnesses associated with fevers can markedly elevate the temperature of the person at the time of death, while chronic illness, dehydration, or the presence of prolonged shock may lower initial body temperature. There is also some diurnal (basically morning versus evening) variation in body temperature in most people. All this means that the calculation begins with some degree of error.

A dead body looses heat passively by three distinct mechanisms: radiation (heat lost as infrared heat rays), conduction (heat passed on to any object that contacts the body), and convection (heat lost into the moving air). The state of the corpse and the environmental conditions greatly affect the rate of heat loss.

Obesity, heavy clothing, warm still air, exposure to direct sunlight, and an enclosed environment slow heat loss. Fat and clothing make good insulators, so an obese person in a sweater will lose heat much more slowly than would a thin, unclothed corpse exposed to cold or moving air, water, or shade. Children and the elderly tend to lose heat faster, as do those who are chronically ill or emaciated. If the body is in contact with cold surfaces such as marble or cool concrete, heat loss will be greater.

There's still one more curve ball: Several days after death, as fly maggots begin to feed on the corpse, their activity and internal metabolic processes can at times raise the temperature of the corpse. This should not be a problem for the forensic investigator, though, because once this insect activity is that far advanced body temperature is no longer of use.

As you can see, heat loss is fraught with inaccuracies. Still, with early and careful measurement of the core body temperature and consideration for the conditions surrounding the corpse, a reasonably accurate estimate can often be made.

Let's say two people are murdered in a home in New Delhi, during late summer. The bodies are discovered four hours after death. One body is left in the garage where the ambient temperature is 110 degrees Fahrenheit, while the other is in the living room where air conditioning holds the temperature at 72. The corpse inside would lose heat at about 1.5 degrees per hour, so that if the medical examiner had evidence that the death had occurred four hours earlier, he would expect to find a core body temperature of approximately 92 to 93 degrees.

1.5 degrees / hour x 4 hours = 6 degrees

98.6 – 6 = 92.6

If he found a different core temperature, he would revise his estimate. But what if the victim were very old or young, thin, unclothed, or lying on a cold tile floor near an air conditioning vent? Under these circumstances, the heat loss would be more rapid. The core temperature could be 88 to 90 degrees, perhaps even less. If the medical examiner failed to consider these mitigating factors, an erroneous estimate of the time of death could result. For example, if the core temperature was 88 degrees and he failed to adjust for the environmental conditions around the body, he could estimate that approximately seven hours had elapsed since death.

98.6 – 88 = 10.6 / 1.5 = 7.1 hours

An estimate of six to eight hours is quite different from an estimate of three to five hours. The killer may have an iron clad alibi for the former time period, and easily could since he hadn't arrived at the crime scene at that time. He could have been having lunch with twenty people. But only four hours later, he might not have such an alibi.

What of the body in the garage? The experts would expect the corpse to gain heat at the same rate of 1.5 degrees per hour. Thus, the core temperature should be approximately 104 degrees Fahrenheit, or perhaps even higher.

c. Chemical Method: Schourup's formula for the determination of the time of death of any cadaver whose cerebrospinal fluid is examined for the concentration of lactic acid (L.A.), non-protein nitrogen (N.P.N.) and amino acid (A.A.), and whose axillary's temperature has been taken at the time the cerebrospinal fluid has been removed.

To make an approximate estimate of the duration of death from the body temperature, the Schourup's formula has been suggested;

$$36 - T + \text{antilog}, \underline{L.A.} + \underline{N.P.N. - 15} + \underline{A.A - 1} \;\; \underline{180 - 16.7 - 7.35}$$
$$4$$

T = Temperature

1 = Axillary's Temperature

The lactic acid content of the cerebro-spinal fluid rises from 15 mg. to 200 mg. per 100cc. The rise is rapid during the first five hours after death. The non-protein nitrogen (N.P.N.) increases from 15mg. to 40mg per 100cc. During the first fifteen hours.

This test is modified by the ante-mortem and rapid cooling of the body. Amino-acides (A.A.) increases from 1 mg. to 12 mg. percent during the first fifteen hours, but the results are modified by rapid cooling of the body.

Limitations of the Schourup's Formula

a. The method is only applicable to adults, as the rate of biochemical change in a child is far more rapid than in adult. It is of value to person over the age of fifteen years.

b. The cerebrospinal fluid must be free of blood, the presence of which raises the lactic concentration.

c. Injuries must not have allowed the escape of cerebrospinal fluid.

d. Death must have occurred within a period of fifteen hours prior to the withdrawal of the sample of cerebrospinal fluid, as after that time the changes in the concentration per time unit becomes irregular.

4. Insesibility and Loss of Power to Move

After death the whole body is insensible. No kind of stimulus is capable of letting the body have voluntary movement. This condition must be observed in conjunction with cessation of heartbeat and circulation and cessation of respiration.

The insensibility and loss of power to move may be present although living, in the following conditions: apoplexy, epilepsy, trance, catalepsy, cerebral concussion, and hysteria.

5. Changes in the Skin

a. Discoloration: After death the skin may be observed to be pale and waxy-looking due to the absence of circulation. Areas of the skin especially the most dependent portions will develop livid discoloration on account of the gravitation of blood.

b. Loss of Elasticity of the Skin: Normally when the body surface is compressed, it readily returns to normal shape. After death, application of pressure to the skin surface will make the surface flattened. Application of pressure with the fingertip will produce impression, like one observed in edema.

On account of the loss of elasticity of the skin and of the post- mortem flaccidity of muscles, the body becomes flattened over areas that are in contract with the surface it rest, and it is called post-mortem contact flattening.

This is observed at the region of the shoulder blades, buttocks, and calves if death occurs while lying on his back. Certain degree of pressure may be applied on the face immediately after death and may be mistaken for traumatic deformity.

c. Opacity of the Skin: Exposure of the hand of a living person to translucent light will allow the red color of circulation to be seen underneath the skin. The skin of a dead person is opaque due to the absence of circulation.

d. Effect of the Application of Heat: Application of melted sealing wax on the breast of a dead person will not produce a blister or inflammatory reaction on the skin. In the living, an inflammatory edema will develop about the wax.

6. Changes in and About the Eye

a. Loss of Corneal Reflex: The cornea is not capable of making any reaction to whatever intensity of light stimulus. However, absence of corneal reflex may also be found in a living person, based on the following conditions: general anesthesia, apoplexy, uremia, epilepsy, narcotic poisoning, and local anesthesia.

b. Clouding of the Cornea: The normal clear and transparent nature of the cornea is lost. The cornea becomes slightly cloudy or opaque after death. If the cornea is kept moist by the application of saline solution after death, it will remain transparent. Opacity of the cornea may be found in certain diseases, like cholera, and therefore is not considered as a reliable sign of death.

c. Flaccidity of the Eyeball: After death, the orbital muscles lose their tone making the intra-orbital tension rapidly fall. The eyeball sinks the orbital fossa. Intra-orbital tension is low.

d. The Pupil is in the Position of Rest: The muscle of the iris loses its tone. The pupil cannot react to light. The size of the pupil varies at the time of death. However, if contracted, it may be found in life in the following conditions: action of drugs like atropine, uremia, tabes dorsails, and apoplexy.

e. The opthalmoscopic findings are as follows:

1. the optic disc is pale and has appearance of optic atrophy, 2. the remaining portion of the fundus may have a yellow tinge which later changes to a brown-gray or slate color, 3. the retina becomes pale like the optic disc, 4. the retinal vessels become segmented, no evidence of blood, and 5. the retinal vessels and arteries are indistinguishable.

f. Tache noir dela sclerotique: After death a spot may be found in the sclera. The spot which may be oval or round or may be triangular with the base towards the cornea and may appear ion the sclera a few hours after death. At the beginning it is yellowish, but later it becomes brown or black. This is believed to be due to the thinning of the sclera thereby making the pigmented choroids visible.

7. Action of Heat on the Skin

This test is useful to determine whether death occurred before or after the application of heat. The heat is applied to a portion of the leg or arm. If death is real, only a dry blister is produced. The epidermis is raised but on prickling the blister, no fluid is present. There is no redness of the surrounding.

In the living, the blister contains abundant serum and area vital reaction-congestion, on the skin is occurred, i.e., loss of animal heat to a point not compatible with life, absence of response of muscle to stimulus, and onset of rigor mortis.

Changes in the Body Following Death

Hereunder are some of early changes in the body following death, as follows:

1. Changes in the Muscle

After death, there is complete relaxation of the whole muscular system. The entire muscular system is contractile for three to six hours after death, and later rigidity sets in. secondary relaxation of the muscles will appear just when decomposition has set in. the following are the stages of the entire muscular tissue after death:

a. Primary Flaccidity or Post-Mortem Muscular Irritability

Immediately after death, there is complete relaxation and softening of all the muscle of the body. The extremities may be flexed, the lower jaw falls, the eyeball loses its tension, and there may incontinence of urination and defecation.

To determine whether the muscles are still irritable, apply electric current and note whether there is still irritability of the muscles. Normally during the stage of primary flaccidity, the muscles are still contractile and react to external stimuli, mechanical or electrical owing to the presence of molecular life after somatic death.

This stage is usually lasts about three to six hours after death. In warm places, the average duration is only one hour and fifty minutes. Chemically, the reaction of the muscle is alkaline and the normal constituents of the individual muscle proteins are the same as life.

b. Post-Mortem Rigidity or Cadaveric Rigidity or Death Stiffening or Death Struggle of the Muscles or Rigor Mortis:

Three to six hours after death the muscles gradually stiffen. It usually starts at the muscles of the neck and lower jaw and spreads downwards to the chest, arms, and lower limbs. Usually the whole body becomes stiff after twelve hours. All the muscles are involved- both voluntary and involuntary. In the heart rigor mortis may be mistaken for cardiac hypertrophy.

Chemically, there is an increase of lactic acid and phosphoric content of the muscle. The reaction becomes acidic. There is no definite explanation as to how such contraction of muscles occurs although it has been proven that there id coagulation of the plasma protein.

In the medico-legal point of view, post-mortem rigidity may be utilized to approximate the length of time the body has been dead. In temperate countries it usually appears three to six hours after death, but in warmer countries it may develop earlier.

In temperate countries, rigor mortis may last for two or three days but in tropical countries the usual duration is twenty-four to forty-eight hours during cold weather and eighteen to thirty-six hours during summer. When rigor mortis sets in early, it passes off quickly and vice-versa.

Conditions Stimulating Rigor Mortis

1. Heat Stiffening

If the dead body is exposed to temperature above 75° it will coagulate the muscle protein and cause the muscles to be rigid. The stiffening is more or less permanent and may not be easily affected by putrefaction. The body assumes the pugilistic attitude with the lower and upper extremities flexed and hands clenched because the flexor muscles are stronger than the extensors.

2. Cold Stiffening

The stiffening of the body may be manifested when the body is frozen, but exposure to warm conditions will make such stiffening disappear. The cold stiffening is due to solidification of fat when the body is exposed to freezing temperature. Forcible stretching of the flexed extremities will produce a sound due to the frozen synovial fluid in the elbows and knees.

3. Cadaveric Spasm or Instantaneous Rigor

This is the instantaneous rigidity of the muscles which occurs at the moment of death due to extreme nervous system or injury to the chest. It is principally due to the fact that the last voluntary contraction of muscle during life does not stop after death but is continuous with the act of cadaveric rigidity. In case of cadaveric spasm, a weapon may be held in the hand before death and can be removed with difficulty.

For practical purposes it cannot be possible for the murderer or assailant to imitate the condition. In cadaveric spasm, only group of muscles are involved and they are usually asymmetrical. The findings of weapon, hair, pieces of clothing, weeds on the palms or even firearms in the hands, and firmly grasped by the victim are very important medico- legal point in the determination whether it is case of suicide, murder or homicide.

The presence of weeds held by the hands of a person found in water shows that the victim was alive before disposal. Instantaneous rigor may also be found following the ingestion of cyanide but usually it is generalized and symmetrical. Strychnine may produce the same, but rigidity may appears sometime after ingestion.

Rigor Mortis vs. Cadaveric Spasm

1. Time of Appearance

Rigor mortis appears three to six hours after death, while cadaveric spasm appears immediately after death. Rigor mortis is a natural phenomenon, while livor mortis is situational.

2. Muscles Involved

Rigor mortis involves all the muscles of the body whether voluntary or involuntary, while cadaveric spasm involves only a certain muscle or group of muscles and are asymmetrical, and that is rigid from farthest part away from the body and less rigid closer to the body.

3. Occurrence

Rigor mortis is a natural phenomenon which occurs after death, while cadaveric spasm may or may not appear on a person at the time of death.

4. Medico-Legal Significance

Rigor mortis may be utilized by medical jurists to approximate the time of death, while cadaveric spasm may be useful to determine the nature of crime.

c. Secondary Flaccidity or Secondary Relaxation

After the disappearance of rigor mortis, the muscle becomes soft and flaccid. It does not respond to mechanical or electrical stimulus. This is due to the dissolution of the muscle proteins which have previously been coagulated during the period of rigor mortis.

The body while at the stage of rigor mortis, if stretched or flexed to become soft will no longer be rigid. This condition of the muscles is not considered as a secondary flaccidity.

2. Changes in Blood

a. Coagulation of the Blood

The stasis of the blood due to cessation of circulation enhances the coagulation of blood inside the blood vessels. The clotting of the blood is accelerated in cases of death by infectious fevers and delayed in cases of asphyxia, poisoning by opium, hydrocyanic acid or carbon monoxide poisoning.

Ante-Mortem vs. Post-Mortem Clot

Ante-Mortem Clot	**Post-Mortem Clot**
1. Firm consistency.	1. Soft in consistency
2. Surface of the blood vessels raw after the blood is removed.	2. Surface of the blood vessel clots are smooth and healthy after clots are removed.
3. Clot homogenous in construction so it cannot be stripped into layer.	3. Clots can be stripped into layer
4. Clots with uniform color.	4. Clots with distinct layer.

The clothing of blood is very slow process that there is a tendency for the blood to separate forming a red clot at the lower level and above it is a while clot known as chicken-fat clot. Blood may remain fluid inside the blood vessels after death.

b. Post-mortem Lividity or Cadaveric Lividity or Post-Mortem Suggillation or Post Mortem Hypostasis or Livor Mortis

The stoppage of the heart action and the loss of tone of blood vessels cause the blood to be under the influence of gravity. Blood begins to accumulate in the most dependent portions of the body. The capillaries may be distended with blood. The distended capillaries coalesce with one another until the whole area becomes dull-red or purplish in color known as post-mortem lividity. If the body is lying on his back, the lividity will develop on the back.

Areas of bone prominence may not show lividity on account of the pressure. If the position of the body is moved during early stage of its formation, it may disappear and develop again in the most dependent area in new position assumed. But if the position of the body has been changed after clotting or the blood has set in or when blood has already diffused into the tissue of the body, a change of position of the body will not alter the location of the post-mortem lividity.

Ordinarily, the color of post-mortem lividity is dull-red or pink or purplish in color, but in death due to carbon monoxide poisoning, it is bright pink. Exposure of the dead body to cold or hot may cause post- mortem lividity to be bright-red in color. The lividity usually appears three to six hours after death and the condition increases until blood coagulates. The time of its formation is accelerated in cases of death due to cholera, uremia and typhus fever. Twelve hours after death, the post-mortem lividity is already fully developed. This also involves all the internal organs.

Characteristics of Post-Mortem Lividity

1. It occurs in the most extensive areas of the most dependent portions of the body.
2. It only involves the superficial layer of the skin.
3. It does not appear elevated from the rest of the skin.

4. The color is uniform, but the color may become greenish at the start of the decomposition.
5. There is no injury of the skin.

Kinds of Post-Mortem or Cadaveric Lividity

1. Hypostasis Lividity

The blood merely gravitates into the most dependent portions of the body but still inside the blood vessels and till fluid in form. Any change of position of the body leads to the formation of the lividity in another place. This occurs in another during the early stage of its formation.

2. Diffusion Lividity

This appears during the later stage of its formation when the blood has coagulated inside the blood vessels or has diffused into the tissues of the body. Any change of position will not change the location of the lividity.

Importance of Cadaveric Lividity

1. It is one of the signs of death; and the color of lividity may indicate the cause of death and even the cause of death if there are changes in its color.
2. It may determine whether the position of the body has been changed after its appearance in the body.
3. It may determine how long the person has been dead; and it gives the investigator and medico-legal examiners an idea as to the time of death.

Considerations in the Position of the Body

1. Posture of the Body When Found

The body may become rigid in the position in which he died. Post- mortem lividity may develop in the assumed position. This condition may occur and is of value if the state and position of the body was not moved before rigidity and lividity took place.

2. Post-Mortem Hypostasis or Lividity

Hypostatis lividity will be found in areas of the body which comes in contact with the surface where the body lies. If there is already coagulation of blood or if blood has already diffused into the tissues of the body, a change of position will not after the location of the post-mortem lividity.

3. Cadaveric Spasm

In violent death, the attitude of parts of the body may infer position on account of the same muscles.

4. Autolytic or Autodigestive Changes after Death

After death, protoelytic, glycolytic and lipolytic ferments of glandular tissues continue to act which lead to the auto digestion of organs. This action is facilitated by weak acid and higher temperature. It is delayed by the alkaline reaction of the tissues of the body and low temperature in the surrounding environment.

Their early appearance is observed in the parenchymatous and glandular tissues. Autolytic action is seen in the maceration of the dead fetus inside the uterus. The stomach may be perforated, glandular tissues become soft after death due to autodigestion and the action of autolytic enzymes.

Microscopic examination of the tissues under the influence of autolytic enzymes shows disintegration, swelling or shrinkage, vacuolization and formation of small granules within the cytoplasm of the cells. There is also a change in the staining capacity and become desquamated from the underlying layers.

5. Putrefaction of the Body

Putrefaction is the breaking down of the complex protein into simpler components associated with the evolution of foul smelling **gassdes** and accompanied by the change of color of the body.

Tissue Changes in Putrefaction

The following are the principal changes undergone by the soft tissues of the body after putrefaction.

1. Changes in the Color of the Tissues

A few hours after death, there is hemolysis of the blood within blood vessels, and as a result of which hemoglobin is liberated. The hemoglobin diffuses through the wall of the blood vessels and stains the surrounding tissues thereby imparting a red or reddish-brown color.

While in the tissues, the hemoglobin undergone chemical changes and various derivatives of hemoglobin are formed. On account of these chemical changes the tissue is gradually changed to greenish-yellow, greenish-blue, or greenish –black color.

The earliest change is greenish in color of the skin that can be seen at the region of the right iliac fossa, and it gradually spreads over the whole abdominal wall. Blood later extravasates into the cavities of the body.

The prominence of the superficial veins with reddish discoloration during the process of decomposition that develops on both flanks of the abdomen, root of the neck and shoulder and which makes the area look like a marbled reticule of branching vein. This is observed easily among the dead persons with fair complexion, and this is simply called as marbolization.

2. Evolution of Gases in the Tissues

One of the byproducts of putrefaction is the evolution of gases. Carbon dioxide, ammonia, hydrogen, sulphurated hydrogen, phosporetted hydrogen, and methane gasses are formed. The offensive odor is due to these gases, and also due to a small quantity of mercaptans.

The formation of gasses causes the distention of the abdomen and bloating of the whole body. Gases formed in the subcutaneous tissues and in the face and neck cause swelling of the whole body. Small gas bubbles are found in the solid visceral organs and give rise to the foamy appearance of the organs.

Effects of Gases on Putrefaction

1. Displacement of the Blood

There may be post-mortem bleeding in open wounds on account of the increased pressure inside the body brought about the accumulation of gases. The lividity may be shifted to other parts of the body.

2. Bloating of the Body

On account of the accumulation of gas, the body is blown-up and swollen. The eyes may be protruding from it sockets, the tongue may come out of the mouth, and the face is black with thick lips having the appearance of a Negro or tete de negri.

3. Fluid Coming Out of Nostrils and Mouth

Fluid coming out of both nostrils and mouth is usually in the form of froth. It is due to the putrefaction of the upper gastro-intestinal and respiratory tracts.

4. Extrusion of the Festus in Gravid Uterus

On account of the increased intra-abdominal pressure, the contents of the gravid uterus may expelled, but this event is quite doubtful when the product of conception is nearing full terms because of the difficulty of expulsion. There is more likehood for the uterus to rupture inside the abdominal cavity.

5. Floating of the Body

The specific gravity of a decomposed body is much less as compared with recently dead. This is due to the increase of gaseous content and increase in volume due to bloating without any increase in weight.

6. Liquefaction of the Soft Tissues

As decomposition progresses, the soft tissues of the body undergo softening and liquefaction. The eyeballs, brain, stomach, intestine, liver and spleen putrefy rapidly, while highly muscular organs and tissues relatively putrefy late.

Factors Modifying the Rate of Putrefaction

1. Internal Factor

a. Age: healthy bodies decompose later than infants. It may be late in a newborn infant who has not yet been fed. Markedly emaciated person has the tendency to mummify.

b. Condition of the body: Those of the full-grown and highly obese persons decompose more rapidly than skinny ones. Bodies of still born are usually sterile so decomposition is retarded.

c. Cause of death: Bodies of person whose cause of death is due to infection decompose rapidly. This is also true when the diseased condition is accompanied with anasacra.

2. *External Factors*

a. Free air: The accessibility of the body to free air will hasten decomposition.

b. Condition of the air: Is loaded with septic bacteria, decomposition will be hastened.

c. Moderate moisture: Moderate amount of moisture will accelerate decomposition, but excessive amount will prevent the access of air to the body thereby delaying decomposition. Moisture is necessary for the growth of and multiplication of bacteria, however, if the evaporation of fluid is marked, there will be mummification of the tissues and putrefaction will be retarded.

d. Temperature of the air: The optimum temperature for specific decomposition is 70°F to 100°F. Decomposition does not occur at temperature below 32°F or about 21°F.

e. Light: The organism responsible for the putrefaction prefers more on the absence of light.

f. Earth: Dry absorbent soil retards decomposition, while most fertile soil accelerates decomposition.

g. Water: Decomposition in running water is more rapid than in still water. Bacteria-laden pools will accelerate decomposition.

h. Clothing: Clothing initially hastens putrefaction by maintaining body temperature but in the later stage, clothing delay decomposition by protecting the body from the ravages of flies and other insects. Tight clothing delay putrefaction due to the diminution of blood in the area on account of pressure.

Changes of the Body During Putrefaction

Here are some of the visible changes of the body during putrefaction:

1. External Changes

a. Greenish discoloration over the iliac fossa appearing after one to three days.

b. Extension of the greenish discoloration over the whole abdomen and other parts of the body.

c. Marked discoloration and swelling of the face with bloody froth coming out of the nostrils and mouth.

d. Swelling and discoloration of the scrotum or of the vulva of male and female, respectively.

e. Distention of the abdomen with gases.

f. Development of the bullae and denudation of large irregular surfaces due to the shedding of the epidermis.

g. Bursting of the bullae and denudation of large irregular surfaces due to the shedding of the epidermis.

h. Escape of blood-stained fluid coming from the mouth and nostrils.

i. Brownish discoloration of the surface veins giving an arborescent pattern on the skin.

j. Liquefaction of the eyeballs.

k. Increased discoloration of the body, and progressive increase of abdominal distention.

l. Presence of maggots.

m. Shedding of the nails and loosening of hair.

n. Conversion of the tissue into semi-fluid mass.

o. Facial feature unrecognizable.

p. Bursting of the abdomen and thoratic cavities.

q. Progressive dissolution of the body.

2. Internal Changes

a. Those which putrefy early are as follows: brain lining of the trachea and laryns, stomach and intestines, spleen, liver, and uterus, if pregnant or in purpal stage.

b. Those which putrefy later, are as follows: esophagus, diaphragm, heart, lungs, kidneys, and urinary bladder.

Factors Influencing Changes in the Body

1. State of the Body before Death:

An emaciated person at the time of death will decompose slower as compared with well-nourished individual when placed under the same conditions and circumstances. Skinny person has more tendencies to mummify, especially at the regions of the extremities.

2. Death, Burial and Environment of the Body:

If the temperature of the surroundings at the time of death is conductive for the growth and multiplication of bacteria, them the longer the time such body is exposed to such condition the faster is the decomposition.

However, if the body has been frozen to death for quite a time, there will be retardation of body decomposition. The presence of filthy, pultaceous and organic material in the surroundings coupled with the presence of light and optimum temperature will enhance the decomposition.

3. Effect of Coffin:

The use of coffin will delay decomposition if it is airtight and hard. If soft and weak, water can easily percolate at the floor and top, thus it will not serve the purpose. The body in a coffin usually only the ground.

4. Clothing and Any Covering on the Body:

Clothing and other body covering delay the decomposition. Most often the covered portions of the body are well preserved for sometimes. The most probable reasons why clothing retard decompositions are: a) if affords some protection from insects and aids adipocere formation keeping the body under it continuously moist by absorbing water from the soil. b) the pressure of the clothing of the body.

5. Depth at Which the Body was Buried:

As a general rule, the greater the depth the body has been buried, the better is the preservation. There is aeration in shallow grayed, and this is conducive invitation for insects and other animals. The change of temperature of the body on account of changing weather conditions is more marked in shallow graves.

6. Condition and Type of Soil:

Dry, arid and sandy soil promotes mummiûcation of the body. The presence of straw other organic matters that will introduce more bacteria will accelerate decomposition.

7. Inclusion of Something in the Grave:

Some organic materials, like food are sometimes included with the dead body inside the coffin because of their superstition that it will be utilized by the departed soul in its life hereafter. Its presence inside the coffin will accelerate putrefaction.

8. Access of Air to the Body after Burial:

Air may hasten evaporation of the body fluid and promotes mummiûcation. Bacteria-laden air will promote decomposition. "Humid air will enhance adipocere formation. However, accessibility of air means accessibility of insects and other scavengers that will promote destruction of the soft tissues of the body.

9. Mass grave:

This is seldom seen, except in mass massacre, war and in plane crash. There is relatively rapid and early decomposition of the dead bodies.

10. Trauma of the Body:

Persons -dying from infection decompose rapidly while-those dying of violent death decompose relatively-slow.

Duration of Death

In the determination as to "how long a person has been dead from the condition of the cadaver and other external evidences, the following points must be taken into considerations.

1. Presence of Rigor Mortis

In Warm countries like in India, rigor mortis sets from 2 to 3 hours after death. It is fully developed in the body after 12 hours. It may last from 18 hours to 36 hours and its disappearance is concomitant with the onset of putrefaction.

2. Presence of Post-Mortem Lividity

Post-mortem lividity usually develops to 6 hours-after death. It first appears as a small petechia-like red spots which later coalesce with each other to involve bigger -areas in the most dependent portions of the body, and which is depending upon the position assumed by the body at the time of death.

3. Onset of Decomposition

In India like other tropical countries, decomposition is early, and the average time is 24 to 48 hours after death. It is manifested by the presence of watery, foul-smelling froth coming out of the nostrils and mouth, softness of the body and presence of crepitation when pressure is applied on the skin.

4. Stage of Decomposition

The approximate time of death may be inferred from the degree of decomposition, although it must be made with extreme caution. There are several factors and conditions which modify the putrefaction of the dead body.

5. Entomology of the Cadaver

In order to approximate the time of death by the use of the ûies present in the cadaver, it is necessary to know the life cycle of the ûies. The common ûies undergo larval, pupal and adult stages. The usual time for the egg to be hatched into larva is 24 hours, so that by the mere fact that there are maggots in the cadaver, one can conclude that death has occurred more than 24 hours.

6. Stage of Digestion of Food in the Stomach

It takes normally 3 to 4 hours for the stomach to evacuate its content after meal. The approximate time of death may be deduced from the amount of food in" the stomach in relation to his last meal. This determination is dependent upon the amount of food taken and the degree of tonicity of the stomach.

a. *Size of the Last Meal:* The stomach usually start to empty within ten minutes after the first mouthful has entered. A light, meals leaves the stomach within 1 and 1/2 to 2 hours after being eaten. A medium-sized meal will require 3 to 4 hours. A heavy meal is entirely expelled into duodenum in 4 to 6 hours.

b. *Kind of Meal:* Liquid move more rapidly than semi-solid and later more rapidly than solids.

c. *Personal Variation:* Psychogenic pylorospasm can prevent departure of the meal from a stomach for several hours, contrarywise, a hypermotile stomach may enhance entry, of food into the duodenum.

d. *Kind of Food Eaten:* Vegetables may require more time for gastric digestion. The less fragmentation of the food will require more time to stay in the stomach. The absence or insufûciency of the gastric hydrocliloric acid content and lesser amount of liquid consumed with solid food will likewise delay gastric evacuation.

7. *Presence of Live Flea in the Clothing in Drowning*

A flea can only survive for approximately 24 hours submerged in water. It can no longer be revived if submerged more than that period. In temperate countries, people wear woolen clothes. If the body is found in water, the ûea may be found in the woolen clothing.

The flea recovered must be placed in a watch glass and observed if it is still living. If the ûea still could move, then the body has been in water for a period less than 24 hours. Revival of the life of the ûea is not possible if they are in water for more than 24 hours.

8. *Amount of Urine in the Bladder*

The amount of urine in the urinary bladder may indicate the -time of death when taken into considerations, the last time the victim seen voiding his urine. There are several factors which may modify urination so it must be utilized with cautions.

9. State of the Clothing

A circumstantial proof of the time of death is the apparel of the deceased. If the victim is wearing street clothes, there is more likelihood that death took place at daytime, but if in night gown or pajama, it is more probable that death occurred at night time.

10. Chemical changes in the cerebro-spinal fluid fifteen hours after death, such as:

1. lactic acid increase from 15 mg. to 200 mg. per 100 cc., 2. non-protein nitrogen increase from 15 mg. to 40 mg., and 3. amino-acid concentration rises from 1% to 12% following death.

11. Post-Mortem Clotting and Decoagulation of Blood

Blood clots inside the blood vessels in 6 hours to 8 hours after death. Decoagulation of blood occurs at the early stage of decomposition.

The presence of any of these conditions may infer the approximate duration of death.

12. Presence or Absence of Soft Tissues in Remains

Under ordinary condition, the soft tissues of the body may disappear. The disappearance of the soft tissues varies and influenced by several factors. When the body is found on the surface of the ground, aside from the natural forces of nature responsible for the destruction of the soft tissues, external element and animals may accelerate its destruction.

13. Conditions of the Bone

If all the soft tissues have already disappeared from the skeletal remains, the degree of erosion of the epiphyseal ends of long bones, pulverization of ûat bones and diminution of weight due to the loss of animal matter may be the basis of the approximation.

Value of Medico-Legal Aspects of Death

Medical expertise is crucial in death investigations. It begins with body examination and evidence collection at the scene and proceeds through history, physical examination, laboratory tests, and diagnosis in short, the broad ingredients of a doctor's treatment of a living patient. The key goal is to provide objective evidence of cause, timing, and manner of death for adjudication by the criminal justice system.

Death investigations carry broad- societal importance for criminal justice and public health. Death investigations provide evidence to convict the guilty and protect the innocent, whether they are accused of murder, child maltreatment, neglect, or other crimes. Death investigations aid civil litigation, such as in malpractice, personal injury, or life insurance claims.

Death investigations are critical for many aspects of public health practice and research, including surveillance, epidemiology, and prevention programs, most often in injury prevention and control but also in prevention of suicide violence, or substance abuse. The value of medico-legal aspects of death is apparent in the screening process. In one county, for example, 8,000 cases are reported to the medical examiner's office, but only 2,000 are accepted.

Screening, which eliminates three-fourths of potential cases, must be handled in a scientifically defensible manner by people with medical training, knowledge, and objectivity. Similarly, ordinary physician do not autopsy burned bodies, but a medical examiner would investigate the possibility of homicide masked as an accident. By interviewing, the medical examiner might uncover evidence of a crime. A" medico-legal examiner brings important skills to the interview of next of kin and others who provide a medical history.

4

Investigation of Death

The sudden or unexplained death of an individual has a profound impact on families and friends of the deceased and places significant responsibility on the police or law enforcement agencies and medico-legal agencies tasked in determining the cause -of death of the victim. Increasingly, the advent of science and technology play a key role in death investigations.

A competent and thorough death scene investigation provides the basis for comprehensive medico-legal inquiries, and together with the crime scene investigations and autopsy examinations provide the basis for an accurate determination helps assure that all relevant aspects of all deaths are fully investigated.

Stages of Medico-Legal Investigation of Death

Hereunder are the different stages of medico-legal investigation of death:

1. Crime Scene Investigation

The crime scene is the place where the essential ingredients of the criminal act took place. It includes the setting of the crime and also the adjoining places of entry and exit of both offender and victim. Not all crimes have a well-defined scene, like estafa(certain forms of swindling), malversation, continuing crimes, etc. However where medical evidence may be present, like murder, homicide, physical injuries, sex crime, crime scene is almost invariability present.

Crime scene investigation includes appreciation of its condition and drawing of inference from it. It also includes the collection of the physical evidences that may lead to the identity of the perpetrator, the manner the criminal act was executed, and such other things that may be useful in the prosecution of the case. There are five methods of crime scene search, i.e., strip search, double strip search or grid method spiral method, wheel method, and zone method.

2. Autopsies

An autopsy is a comprehensive study of a dead body, performed by a trained physician employing recognized dissection procedure and techniques. It includes removal of tissues for further examination. There are two kinds of, autopsies, i.e., hospital or non-official autopsy, and medico-legal or official autopsy.

a. Hospital or Non-Official Autopsy

This is-an autopsy done on a human body with the consent of the deceased person's relatives for the purpose of, i.e., determining the cause of death; providing correlation of clinical diagnosis and clinical symptoms; determining the effectiveness of therapy; studying the natural cause of disease process and educating students and physicians.

b. Medico-Legal or Official-Examination

This is the purpose of determining the cause, mode, and time of death; recovering, identifying, and preserving evidentiary material; providing interpretation and correlation of facts and circumstances related to death; providing a factual, objective medical report for law enforcement, prosecution, and defense agencies; and separating death due to disease from death due to external cause for protection of the innocent.

Pathological vs. Medico-Legal Autopsies

Hereunder are the distinctions between pathological and medico-legal aspects of autopsies.

Aspect	Pathological	Medico-Legal
1. Requirement	Must have the consent of the next of kin.	It is the law that it gives the consent.

2. Purpose	Confirmation of the clinical findings to the criminal act.	Correlation of changes to the research.
3. Emphasis	Notation of all the all abnormal findings.	Emphasis laid on the effect of the wrongful act to the body. Other findings may only be noted in mitigation of the criminal responsibility
4. Conclusion	Summation of all abnormal findings irrespective of its correlation with clinical findings.	Must be specific for the purpose of determing whether it is in relation to the criminal act.
5. Minor or Pathological	Need not be mentioned in the report	If the investigator think it will be useful in the administration of justice, then it must be included.

4. Conclusion

Summation of all abnormal findings irrespective of its correlation with clinical findings. It is the law that it gives the consent.

Correlation of Changes to the Criminal Act

Emphasis laid on the effect of the wrongful act to the body. Other findings may only be noted in mitigation of the criminal responsibility Must be specific for the purpose of determining whet-her it is in relation to the criminal act.

5. Minor or Pathological Need not be mentioned in the report

If the investigator think it will be useful in the administration of justice, then it must be included.

Features Peculiar to Medico-Legal Autopsies

1. Clinical history of the deceased in most instances absent, sketchy or doubtful; and the identity of the deceased is the responsibility of the forensic pathologist.

2. A careful examination of the external; surface for possible trauma including the clothing to determine the pattern of injuries in relation to the injurious agent.
3. The autopsy is written in a style that will make it easier for laymen to read and more clearly organized insofar as the mechanism of death is concerned.
4. The time of death, and the timing of tissue injuries must be answered by the forensic pathologist; and the forensic pathologist must alert himself of the possible inconsistencies between the apparent cause of death and his actual findings in the crime scene.
5. The professional and environmental climate of a forensic pathologist is with the courts, attorneys and police who make scrutiny of the ûndings and conclusion.

Guidelines in the Performance of Autopsies

Hereunder are the guidelines in the procedure of autopsies:

1. Be it an official or non-official autopsy, the pathologist must be properly guided by the purpose for which autopsy is to be performed doing the purpose of such dissection will be served.
2. The autopsy must be comprehensive and must not leave some part of the body unexamined. Even if the findings are already sufficient to account of the death, these should not be a sufficient reason for the pre-mature termination of the autopsy. The existence of a certain disease or injury does not exclude the possibility of another much more fatal disease or injury. The finding of coronary disease does not exclude the probability of injury or poisoning.
3. Bodies which are severely mutilated, decomposing or damaged by ûre are still suitable for autopsy. No matter how putrid or fragmentary the remains are, careful examination may be productive of information that bears the identity and other physical trauma received. Frequently a pathologist's reluctance to perform an autopsy on decomposed' body is due to the odor or vermin rather than to his belief that the examination would be productive.

4. All autopsies must be performed in a manner which shows respect of the dead body. Unnecessary dissection must be avoided.
5. Proper identity of the deceased autopsied must be established in non- official autopsy. Autopsy on wrong body may be ground for damages.
6. A dead body must not be embalmed before the autopsy. The embalming fluid. may render the tissue and -blood unfit for toxicological analyses. The embalming may later the gross appearance of the tissues or might results to a wide variety of artifacts that tend to destroy or obscure evidence. Embalmer who applied embalming fluid on a dead body which in its very nature is a victim of violence is liable for his wrongful act.
7. The dead body must be autopsied in the same condition when found at the crime scene. A delay in its performance may fail or modify the possible findings thereby not serving the best interest of justice.

Precautions in Post-Mortem Examination

The following are some of the precautions to be observed, in the conduct of post-mortem examination:

1. The physician must hail all the necessary permit or authorization to perform such an examination. Such permit must be issued by the inquest officer. The absence of such authorization may hold the physician civilly and criminally liable.
2. The physician must have a detailed history of the previous symptoms and condition of deceased to be used as his guide in the post-mortem examination.
3. The true identity of the deceased must be ascertained. If no one claims the body, a complete data to reveal his identity must be taken.
4. Examination must be made in a well-lighted place and it is advisable that to unauthorized persons" should be present.

5. All external findings must be properly described and if possible a sketch must be made or photograph must be taken to preserve the evidence; and all steps and findings in the examination must be recorded.

Stages in the Post-Mortem Examination

Enumerated hereunder the stages in the post-mortem examination of the dead body:

1. Preliminary Examination

a. Examination of the surroundings attention must be focused on the furniture; bullet holes on the ceiling, floor and walls; amount, color and degree of spread of the blood stains, position of the wounding weapon; food and fingerprints and hair and clothes.

b. Examination of the clothing - look for marks to establish identity, kind and quality of the garment, stains, grease, cut and tear or other marks of resistance and violence.

c. Identity of the body - determine the height, weight, color of hair and eyes, complexion, condition and number of teeth, bodily deformity, scars and tattoo marks, clothing, dog tag and fingerprint.

2. External Examination

a. Examination of the body surfaces -inspect the natural oriûce of the body.

All wounds must be described in detail, blood stains and foreign bodies.

b. Determination of the position and approximate time of death in this stage, the presence and degree of hypostasis, rigor mortis and putrefaction and color of the blood stain must be noted. Examination of the hands for the presence of -cadaveric spasm and wounding weapon or any articles may be necessary for the proper solution of the crime under investigation.

c. Internal examination; examine all body oriûces for blood and foreign bodies. Blood coming out of the nostrils may imply fracture on the base of the anterior cranial fossa. Hemorrhage of the ears may imply fracture of the middle cranial fossa.

Mistakes in Medico-Legal Autopsies

Hereunder are some of the mistakes in the conduct of medico-legal autopsies:

1. Errors-or omission in the collection of evidence for identification; failure to make frontal, oblique and proûle photographed of the face; and failure to have ûngerprints made; and failure to have a complete dental examination performed.
2. Errors or omission in the collection or evidence required for establishing the time of death; failure to report the rectal-temperature of the body; failure to observe the changes that may occur in the intensity and distribution of rigor mortis before, during, and after autopsy; and failure to observe the ingredients of the last meal and its location in the alimentary tract.
3. Errors or omission in the collection of evidence required for other medico- legal examination:

a. Failure to collect specimen of blood for determination of the contents of alcohol and barbiturates; and failure to determine the blood group of the dead person if death by violence was associated with external bleeding;

b. Failure to collect nail scrapings and samples of hair if there is reasonable chance that death resulted from assault; and failure to search for seminal fluid if there is a reasonable chance that the fatal injuries had occurred incidental to a sexual crime;

c. Failure to examine clothing; skin and the superûcial portion of the bullet trace for residue of powder, and the failure to collect samples of any residue for the purpose of chemical identification; and failure to use an X- Ray for locating a bullet or fragments of bullet if there is any doubt with regard in their presence and location;

d. Failure to strip the dura mater from the clavaria and base of the skull many-features of the skull have been missed because the pathologist did not expose the surface of the fractional bone; and

e. Failure to protect bullet from defacement, such as likely to occur if there are handled with metal instruments; and failure to collect separate specimens of blood from the right and left sides of the heart in instances in which the body was recovered from water.

4. Errors or omission result in the production of undesirable artifacts or in the destruction of valid evidence:

a. Opening of the skull before blood is permitted to drain form the superior vena cava. If the head is opened before the blood drained from it, blood will almost invariably escape into the subdural and subarachnoid space, and such an observation may then be interpreted as evidence of ante-mortem hemorrhage.

b. The use of a hammer and chisel for opening the skull. A hammer and chisel should never be used for the purpose in a medico-legal autopsy. Fracture produced by the chisel is frequently confused with ante- mortem;

c. Failure to open the thorax under water is one wishes to obtain evidence of pneumothorax; and failure to tie the great vessels between site of transaction and the heart when air embolism is suspected;

d. Failure to open the right ventricle of the heart and the pulmonary artery in situation of pulmonary thrombus-embolism is suspected; and failure to remove the uterus, vagina and vulva en rnase if rape or abortion is suspected.

Causes of Death

The causes of death are injury, disease or combination or both injury and disease responsible for initiating the trend or physiological disturbance, brief or prolonged, which produce the fatal termination. It may be immediate or proximate.

1. Immediate or Primary Cause of Death

This applies to cases when trauma "or disease kill quickly that there is no opportunity for squeal or complications to develop. An extensive brain laceration as a result of a vehicular accident is an example of immediate cause of death.

2. The Proximate or Secondary Cause of Death

The injury or disease was survived for a sufficient prolonged interval which permitted the development of serious squeal which actually caused the death if a stab would in the abdomen later caused generalized peritonis. Therefore, it is conclusive that peritonis is the proximate cause of death.

Medico-Legal Classifications of Death

1. Natural Death

This is death caused by natural disease condition in the body. The disease may develop spontaneously or it might have been a consequence of physical injury inûicted prior to its development. If a natural disease developed without the intervention of the felonious acts of another person, no one can be held responsible for the death.

2. Violent or Unnatural Death

Violent deaths are of those due to injuries inûicted in the body or some forms of outside force. The physical injury must be the proximate cause of death. The death of the victim is presumed to be natural consequence of the physical injuries inflicted, when the following facts are established, i.e., the victim at the time of physical injuries were inûicted was in normal health; the death may be expected from physical injuries inflicted; and ensued within a reasonable time.

Pathological Classification of Death

An analysis of all deaths from natural causes will ultimately lead to the failure of the heart, lungs, and the brain, so that death due to pathological lesions may be classified into:

1. Death from Syncope

This is death due to sudden and fatal cessation of the action of the heart with circulation included.

2. Death from Asphyxia

Asphyxia is a condition in which the supply of the oxygen to the blood or to tissues or to both has reduced below.

3. Death from Coma

Coma is the state of unconsciousness with insensibility of the pupil and conjunctivae, and inability to swallow, resulting from the arrest of the functions of the brain.

Death Scene Investigation

The medico-legal expert and the investigator must do their best to find answers for families who have lost loved ones. Death investigation requires strict adherence to guidelines. Crime scene investigators must search for clues that identify a death as natural, suicide or homicide. In the case of homicide, investigators must carefully collect evidence to help identify suspects.

Introductions at the scene allow the investigator to establish formal contact with other official agency representatives. The investigator must identify the first responder to ascertain if any artifacts or contamination may have been introduced to the death scene. The investigator must work with all key people to ensure command protocol and scene safety prior to his/her entrance into the scene.

Appropriate personnel must make a determination of death prior to the initiation of the death investigation. The confirmation or pronouncement of death determine jurisdictional responsibilities. Photograph the crime scene. Photographs provide detailed corroborating evidence that constructs a system at the scene.

5

Death by Asphyxia

The body creates the need to breathe from the excess carbon dioxide in the lungs; and yet the body has no way to detect the absence of oxygen. Many gases, though non-toxic, are classified as simple asphyxiants in their pure form or in high concentrations -for this very reason. Oxygen deficient atmospheres are-the basis for many single and multiple deaths occurring; hence the need to vent or purge the inert gases from all tanks before entry.

Definition of Asphyxia

Asphyxia is the general term applied to all forms of violent death which results primarily from the interference with the process of respiration or the condition in which the supply of -oxygen to the-blood or to the tissue or both has been reduced below normal level.

Types of Asphyxial Death

Hereunder are the types of asphixial death:

1. Anoxie Death

This is associated with the failure of the arterial blood to become normally saturated with oxygen. It may be due to, i.e., breathing in an atmosphere without or with insufficient oxygen as in high latitude, obstruction of the air passage due to pressure from outside, as in traumatic crush asphyxia; paralysis of the respiratory center due to poisoning injury or anesthesia, etc.

2. Anemic Anoxic Death

This is due to a decreased capacity of the blood to carry oxygen. This condition may be due to, i.e., severe hemorrhage;

poisoning, like carbon monoxide and low haemoglobin level in the blood.

3. Stagnant Anoxic Death

This is brought about by the failure of circulation. The failure of circulation may be due to; heart failure, shock, and arterial and venous obstructions, incident to embolism, vascular spasm, or the use of tourniquet.

4. Histotoxic Anoxic Death

This is due to the failure of the cellular oxidative process, although the oxygen delivered to the tissues, it cannot be utilized properly, cyanide and alcohol are common agents responsible for histotoxic anoxic death.

Phases of Asphyxial Death

The following are the phases of asphyxial death:

1. Dyspneic Phase

The symptoms are due to lack of oxygen and the retention of carbon dioxide in the body tissue. The breathing becomes rapid and deep, the pulse rate increases, and there is a rise in the blood pressure. The face, hands and fingernails become bluish especially in the case of the newly born infants.

2. Convulsive Phase

This is due to the stimulation of the central nervous system by carbon dioxide. The cyanosis becomes more pronounced and the eyes become staring and the pupils are dilated. Examination of the visceral. Organs shows small petechial hemorrhages, commonly known as Tardieu Spot.

The Tardieu Spots are caused by the hemorrhage produced by the rupture of the capillaries on. account of the increase of intra-capillary pressure. It usually appears in place where the tissue is soft rand the capillaries are not well supported by the surroundings, as in visceral organs, skin, conjunctivae, and capsules of glands.

3. Apneic Phase

The apnea is due to paralysis of the respiratory center of the brain. The breathing becomes shallow and gasping and the rate becomes slower till death. The hearth later fails. Recovery at this stage is almost nil due to the permanent damage inside the brain on account of prolonged cerebral anoxia.

Classifications of Asphyxia

Enumerated and discussed hereunder are the most common classifications of asphyxia:

1. Asphyxia by Hanging

Asphyxia by hanging is a form of violent death brought about by the suspension of the body by a ligature which encircles the neck and the constricting force is the weight of the body. It is not necessary that the whole body will be left suspended. The victim may be sitting or lying with the face downward provided that the pressure is present in front or the side of the neck.

2. Asphyxia by Strangulation

Strangulation by ligature is produce by compression of the neck by means of ligature which is tightened by a force other than the weight of the body. Usually, the ligature is drawn by pulling the ends after crossing at the back or front of the neck; or several folds of the ligature may be around the neck tightly placed and the ends are knotted or a loop it thrown over the head and a stick inserted beneath it and twisted till the noose is drawn tight.

If the ligature is made of soft material and is applied smoothly around the neck, no visible mark will be observed after death. Hard rough ligature applied with force more than that required to kill may produce extensive abrasion and contusion at the area of application. Strangulation by ligature may be observed in infanticide using the umbilical cord as the constricting material.

This must be differentiated from accidental strangulation by the umbilical cord during childbirth. In accidental strangulation during child birth, the umbilical cord is abnormally long and there is no disturbance in the wharton's jelly. Strangulation by ligature is commonly observed in rape cases, but the presence of findings in the genitalia and other physical injuries are the distinctive findings.

3. Aspliyxia by Drowning

This is a form of asphyxia wherein the nostrils and the mouth has been submerged in nay watery, viscid or pultaceous fluid for a time to prevent the free entrance of air into the air passage and lungs. It is not necessary that the whole body to be submerged in fluid. It is sufficient for the nostrils and mouth to be under ûuid. Children may be drowned in an ornamental pool or fish pond, and an epileptic or drunk person may found -drowned in a shallow creek.

4. Asphyxia by Irrespirable Gases

This death is due to carbon monoxide or carbonic oxide the silent killer. Carbon monoxide is formed from the incomplete combustion of carbon fuel. The fatal carbon monoxide poisoning usually involves burning of wood oil, coal, kerosene and charcoal used in heating or cooking, or gasoline engines in cars.

The occurrence of symptoms is carbon monoxide poisoning depends on the rapidly or intoxication, ability of the individual to tolerate the lack of oxygen and presence of other depressant drugs, usually alcohol. The main action of carbon monoxide is oxygen deprivation and not its toxic manifestation, so the oxygen deprivation of the tissue is the degree of saturation of hemoglobin with the gas.

Accidental and suicidal death by carbon monoxide is common. Victims may be accidentally imprisoned or deliberately enclosed themselves in a room or garage with motor engine running or slow burning is present. Judicial death execution by gas chamber carbon monoxide is utilized in some foreign countries that cause almost painless death.

5. Asphyxia by Pressure on the Chest

This is a form of asphyxia whereby the free exchange of air on the lungs is prevented by the immobility of the chest and abdomen due to external pressure or crush injury.

6. Asphyxia by Suffocation

Asphyxia by suffocation is exclusion of air from the lungs by closure of air openings or obstruction of the air passageway from the. External openings to the air sucks. There are two kinds:

a. Smothering

This is a form of asphyxial death caused by the closing the external. respiratory orifices, either by the use of hand or by some other means. The nostrils and mouth may be blocked by the introduction of foreign substance, like mud, paper, cloth, etc.

b. Choking

This is a form of suffocation brought about by the impaction of foreign body in the respiratory passage. Most of suffocation by choking is accidental, although it may be utilized in suicide or in homicide. The post mortem-finding in suffocation by choking is the same as other forms of asphyxia plus the presence of the foreign body in the respiratory tract.

6

Medico-Legal Aspects of Injuries

Physical injury is the effect of some forms of stimulus on the body. The effect may only be apparent when the stimulus applied is sufficient to cause injury and the body resistance is great. It may be real when the effect is visible. The effect of the application of stimulus may be immediate or may be delayed. A thrust to the body of a sharp pointed and sharp edge instrument will lead to the immediate production of a stab wound, while a hit by a blunt object may cause the delayed production of a contusion.

Definition of Physical Injuries

Physical injuries also include bodily injuries or bodily harms, is damage or harm caused to the structure or function of the body caused by an outside agent or force, which may be physical or chemical, and either by accident or intentional. A severe and life-threatening injury is referred to as a physical trauma. It is also defined as impairment of physical condition or pain. The following are some of the causes of physical injuries, i.e., physical violence, mechanical pressures, heat or cold, electrical energy, chemical energy, change of atmospheric pressure or barotraumas, radiation, and infection.

Groupings of Physical Injuries

Physical injuries resulted from external force maybe grouped into three categories, as follows:

1. Simple Injury

Simple injury has not been define in law; however, an injury which is neither serious nor extensive but heals rapidly without leaving permanent deformity or disfiguration is a simple injury.

2. Grievous Injury

It is any injury which endangers life or which causes an individual person to be, during the space of twenty days in sever bodily pain or unable to follow his or her ordinary pursuits.

3. Fatal Injury

A fatal injury is one that Causes death immediately or within a short time after its inûiction; and these are wounds involving the heart, big blood vessels; the brain, the upper part of the spinal cord, the stomach, the liver, the spleen, and the intestines.

Injuries Brought About by Violence

The effect of the application of physical violence on a person is the production of wound. A wound is the dissolution of the natural continuity of any tissues of the living body. It is the disruption of the anatomic energy of a tissue of the body.

In several occasions, the word physical injury is used interchangeable with wound. However, the effect of physical violence may not always results to the production of wound, but the wound is always the effect of physical violence.

Vital Reactions

It is the stun total of all reaction of tissue or organ to trauma. The reaction may be observed microscopically. The following are the common reactions of a living tissue to trauma.

1. Rubor

Reduces or congestion of the area due to an increase of blood supply as a part of the reparative mechanism.

2. Calor

Sensation of heat or increase in temperature.

3. Dolor

Pain on account of the involvement in the sensory nerve.

4. Loss of Function

On account of the trauma, the tissue may not be able to function normally. The presence of vital reaction differentiates ante-mortem from post-mortem injury.

In the following instances; vital reactions or changes may not be observed even if injury was inflicted during life:

a. If the physical injuries are inûicted during the agonal state of a living person. The body cells or tissue during the period may have the potential capacity to react to the trauma; and

b. If death is so sudden as not to give the tissues of the body, the chance to react properly. This is commonly observed in deaths due to sudden coronary occlusion.

Classifications of Physical Injuries

The following are the classifications of physical injuries:

1. As to severity

a. Mortal Wound

Wound is caused immediately after inûiction or shortly thereafter that is capable of causing death. Parts of the body where the wounds inûicted are considered mortal, i.e., heart and big blood vessels, brain and upper -portion of the spinal cord; lungs, stomach, liver, spleen and intestine.

b. Non-Mortal Wound

This is a type of wound which is not capable of producing death immediately after inûiction of the external, stimuli or outside force or shortly thereafter.

2. As to the kind of instrument used;

a. Wound brought about by blunt instrument, i.e., contusion hematoma, and lacerated wounds.

b. Wound brought about by sharp instrument; i.e., sharp edged instrument- incised wound, sharp pointed instrument: punctured would, sharp-edged and sharp pointed instrument stab wound.

c. Wound brought about by tearing force lacerated wound.

d. Wound brought about by change of atmospheric pressure barotrauma.

e. Wound brought about by heat or cold; frostbite, burns or scald.

f. Wound brought about by chemical explosion; gunshot or shrapnel wound.
g. Wound brought about by infection.

3. As to the manner of infliction

That is, hit-bolo, blunt instrument, axe; thrust or stab-bayonet, dagger; gunpowder explosion-projectile or shrapnel "wound; and siding or rubbing abrasion.

4. As regards to the depth of the wound

a. Superficial

When the wound involves only the layers of the skin.

b. Deep

When the wound involves the inner structure beyond the layers of the slain.

l) Penetrating

It is one in-which the wounding agent enters the body but did not Come out or the mere piercing of a solid organ or-tissue of the body. Penetrating wound, it is a wound where the dimension of depth and direction is an important factor in its description. It involves the skin of mucous surface and deeper underlying tissues or organs, caused directly by the wounding instrument. Puncture, stab, and gunshot wounds usually belong to this type of wound.

2) Perforating

It is produced when the wounding agent produces communication between the inner and outer portion of the hollow organs. It may also mean piercing or traversing completely a particular part of the body causing communication between the points of u entry and exit of the instrument or substance producing it.

5. As regards to the site of the application

a. Coup injury force

Physical injury which is located at the site of the application of *b. Contre Coup Injury force*

Physical injury found opposite at the site of the application of the

c. Coup Contre-Coup Injury

Physical injury located at the site and also opposite the site of application of force.

d. Locus Minoris Resistencia

Physical injury located not at the site nor opposite the site of the application of force but in some areas offering the least resistance to the force applied. A blow on the forehead may cause contusion at the region of the eyeball because of the fracture on the papyraceous bone forming the roof of the orbit.

e. Extensive Injury

Physical injury involving greater area of the body beyond the site of the application of force. It has not only the wide area" of injury but also the varied types of injury. A fall from a height or a run-over victim of vehicular accident may suffer from multiple fractures, laceration of organs, and all types of skin injuries.

When a stationary head is hit by moving object, there is tendency for the development of contusion on the brain at the site of impact. When the moving head hits a firm, fixed and hard. object, brain contusion may develop at the opposite of the site of impact. A coup, contra-coup location of brain injury may be found a fixed head is hit with a moving object and then falls on another hard object.

6. As to regions or organs of the body

That is, head and neck, injuries in the chest, abdominal injuries, pelvic injuries, and extremities: upper and lower.

7. Special Types of Wounds a. Defense Wound

It is a wound which is the result of a person's instinctive reaction of self-protection. Injuries suffered by a person to avoid or repel potential injury contemplated by the aggressor. A person who is conscious that he is going to be hit by a blunt instrument on the head may raise his flexed forearms over his head, causing injuries to the forearms.

If someone is going to stab another with a sharp instrument the tendency of: the potential victim is to take hold of the instrument thus causing the production of an incised stab wound on the palm.

b. Patterned wound

Wound in the nature and shape of an object or instrument and which infers the object or instrument causing it. Impact on the face of the radiator grill of a car may cause imprint of the radiator grill on face.

A person run over by a wheel of a car, tire marks are shown on the body. Due to hanging, the nature of the abrasion mark on the neck may infer material used. Contusion produced by belt, branch of tree metallic rod etc. may have the shape of the wounding instrument.

c. Self-lnflicted Wound

Self-inflicted wound is a wound produced one oneself. As distinguished from suicide, the person has no intention to end his life.

Motives of Producing Self-Inflicted Wound

1. To escape certain obligations or punishment. During wartime; soldiers may cut their fingers to avoid frontline assignments and prisoners may inflict physical injuries on their body to avoid hard labor and just be confined in a hospital to receive food and rest.
2. To create or deliberately magnify an existing injury or disease for pension of workman's compensation.
3. To create a new identify or destroy the existing one. Fingerprints maybe destroyed by acid, by cutting or burning. A person may even request for the service of a plastic surgeon to create a new identify or destroy existing ones.
4. To gain attention or sympathy, and psychotic behavior.

Some Ways of Self-Mutilation

1. 'Head hanging or bumping, this is commonly observed in overactive children and cause hematoma.
2. Exposure of parts of the body to heat radiation from open fires, radiators, or protective grills over radiator-thermophilia.
3. Penetrating nail or spike to the chest wall or insertion into the urinary bladder in a female.
4. Castration by amputation of the penis.
5. Trauma inûicted on the female genitalia to induce abortion or promotes hemorrhage and creates an anemia.
6. Subcutaneous injection of fecal matters to promote abscess formation.
7. Pricking of acne eruption Ito lead to a severe facial disfigurement.
8. Subcutaneous injection of air which is creating a condition of emphysema.
9. Nail-biting onychopagia, which may lead to maceration of the skin and infection.
10. Grinding of the teeth or bruxism, is frequently seen ill the mentally retarded and can lead to abnormal tooth wear, a bilateral hypertrophy of the masseter and a pain on chewing.
11. Pressure on the subcutaneous tissue by a tightly applied cord or belt around the body, i.e., tribal customs of metal band around neck or a. leg by some Afro-asian tribes may cause permanent disûgurement, and use of shoes made of metal by Chinese women.
12. Pulling of the body hair-tricliotillomania.

Medical Classifications of Wounds

Enumerated hereunder are the different medical classification of wounds:

l. Closed Wounds

There is no breach of continuity of the skin or mucous membrane.

a. Superficial

When the wound is just beneath the layers of the —skin or mucous membrane.

1. Petechiae

This is circumscribed extravasations of the blood in the subcutaneous tissue or underneath the mucous membrane. The cause of passage of blood from capillaries may be due to the increase intra-capillary pressure or increased permeability of the vessel.

The hemorrhage maybe small or pinhead sized but several petechiae may coalesced to form a bigger hemorrhagic area. Mosquito or other insect bites may cause the formation of circumscribed hemorrhages.

Petechiae are not always a product of trauma. Petechial hemorrhage may be a post-mortem in death by hanging. There are; gravitation of blood into the most dependent part of the body which eventually leads to rupture of over distended capillaries seen at the region of the leg.

2. Contusion

Contusion is the effusion of blood into the tissues underneath the skin on account of the rupture of the blood vessels as a result of the application of blunt force or violence. When a blunt force is applied, it momentarily compresses the blood vessels at the point of contact, thereby temporarily forcing the blood out of the area and setting up a fluid wave under pressure.

When the pressure exceeds the cohesive force of the cells forming the capillary, arteriole, or venule wall, the vessel ruptures. Inasmuch as it used to take more time for the blood to get out of the blood vessels, contusion does not immediately develop after the application force. It may develop after a lapse of minutes or even hours after the application force.

The variation depends on the part of the body injured, tenderness of the tissues affected, condition of the blood vessels involved, and natural disease. Women are much more easily bruised than men while boxers are less prone to suffer contusion despite of heavy punishment. The size of the contusion is usually greater than the size of the object causing it.

The location of the contusion may not always indicate the site of the application of the force. For instance, a blow of the forehead may cause black eye or contusion around the tissues of the eye ball, or a thick on the leg may cause appearance of contusion at the region of the ankle on account of the gravitation of the effusion between muscles and fascia.

On the medico-legal viewpoint, a contusion as indicated by its external pattern may correspond to the shape of the object or weapon used to produce it; its extent may suggest the possible degree of violence applied; and its distribution may indicate the character and manner of injury as in manual strangulation around the neck. It may infer grave complications and consequences on account of serious injuries of the underlying tissues.

a. Age of Contusion

The age of contusion can be appreciated from its color changes. The size tends to become smaller from the periphery to the center and passes through a series of color changes as a result of the disintegration of the red blood corpuscles and liberation of hemoglobin.

The contusion is red, sometimes purple soon after its complete development, i.e., in 4 to 5 days, the color changes to green; in 7 to 10 days, it becomes yellow and gradually disappears on the 14th or 15th day; the ultimate disappearance of color varies upon the severity and constitution of the body, and the color changes starts from the periphery inwards.

b. Factors influencing the degree and extent of contusion

The general condition of the victim some healthy persons are easily bruised; part of the body affected bloody parts of the body produce larger contusion, specially where subcutaneous tissue is loose.

In areas of the body with excessive fat, contusion easily develops, while parts of the body with abundant ûbrous tissue and god muscle tone, bruising less; and amount of force applied-other factors being equal, the greater the force applied the more effusion of blood will develop.

The disease contusion may develop with or without the application of force. Examples: purpura, memophilia, aplastic, anemia, whooping cough, even vicarious menstruation.

The age; children and old age persons tend to bruise more easily. Children have loose and tender old persons have less ûesh and the blood vessels are more fragile; sex; woman, especially if obese, easily develop contusion. Athletes, like boxers do not develop contusion easily.

The application of heat and cold if immediately after injury cold. compress is applied, the production of contusion will be minimized. After it has already developed- application of warm compress will hasten disappearance.

The distinction between ante-mortem and post-mortem contusions in an undecomposed body is that in ante-mortem bruising, there is swelling, damage to epithelium, extravasation, coagulation and inûltration of the tissues with blood, while in post-mortem bruising there are no such findings.

3. Hematoma

Hematoma is the extravasations or effusion of blood in a newly formed cavity underneath the skin. It usually develops. when the blunt instrument is applied in part of the body where bony tissues is superûcially located, like the head, chest and the anterior respect of legs.

The force applied causes the sub-cutaneous tissues rupture on account of the presence of a hard structure underneath. The destruction of the sub-cutaneous will lead to the accumulation of blood causing it to elevate.

Contusion vs. Hematoma

a. In contusion the effused blood are in the interstices of the tissue underneath the skin, while the hematoma blood accumulates in a newly formed cavity underneath the skin.

b. In contusion, the skin shows no elevation and if ever" elevated, the elevation is slight and is on account of inûamatory changes while in hematoma the outer layer of the skin is always elevated making it visible to naked eye.

c. In contusion, puncture or aspiration with syringe of the lesion, no blood can be obtained, while in hematoma, aspiration will show presence of blood and subsequent depression of the elevated lesion. Abscess, ûbroid thickening, and even malignancy are potential complications of hematoma.

b. Deep

a. Musculo-Skeletal Injuries

1. Sprain

Partial or complete disruption in the community of a muscular or ligarnentous support of a joint. It is usually caused by a blow kick or torsion force.

2. Dislocation

Displacement of the articular surface of bones entering into the formation of a joint.

3. Fracture

Dissolution of the continuity of bone resulting from violence or some existing pathology.

a. Close or Simple Fracture; fracture wherein -there is no break in continuity of the over-lying skin or where the external air has no point of access to the site of injury.

b. Open or Compound Fracture; the fracture is complicated by an open wound caused by the broken bone which protruded with other tissues of the broken skin

c. Greenstick Fracture; fracture wherein only one side of the bone while the other side is merely bent.

d. Comminuted Fracture; the fractured bone is fragmented into several pieces.

e. Linear Fracture - when -the fracture forms a crack commonly observed flat bones.

f. Subluxation; incomplete or partial dislocation of the bones.
g. Spiral Fracture; the break in the bone form a spiral manner as observed in long bones.
h. Pathologic Fracture; fracture caused by weakness of the bone due to disease rather than violence.
i. Strain; the over-stretching, instead of an actual tearing or the rupture of a muscle or ligament which may not be associated with the joint.

b. Internal Hemorrhage

Rupture of blood vessel which may cause hemorrhage maybe due to the following, i.e., traumatic intracranial hemorrhage, rupture of parenchymatous organs and laceration of other parts of the body.

c. Cerebral Concussion-Commotion Cerebri

Cerebral concussion is the jarring or stunning of the brain characterized by more or less complete suspension of its functions, as a result of injury to the head, which leads to some commotion of the cerebral substance. Cerebral concussion is much more severe when the moving or mobile head struck a fixed object as compared when the head is ûxed and struck by a hard object loving.

Signs and Symptoms of Concussion

1. Unconsciousness which is more or less complete.
2. Muscles relaxed and ûaccid.
3. Eyelids are closed and the conjuctivae are insensitive.
4. Surface of the body is pale, cold and clammy.
5. Respiration is slow, shallow and hanging.
6. Temperature is sub-normal.
7. Pulse is rapid, weak, faltering and scarcely perceptible to the fingers.
8. Sphincters are relaxed perhaps with unconscious evacuation of the bowel and bladder.

9. Reflexes are present but sluggish and in severe cases may be absent. Loss of memory for events just before the injury retrograde anmesia, is a constant effect of cerebral concussion and its medico-legal importance.

2. *Open Wound;*

There is a breach of continuity of the skin or mucous membrane, viz., Abrasion, Scratch, Graze and Friction Mark. It is an injury characterized by the removal of the superficial epithelial layer of the skin caused by a rub or friction against a hard rough surface. Whenever, there is forcible contact before friction occurs. There may be contusion associated with abrasion, The shape varies and the raw surface exudes blood and lymph which later dries and forms a protective covering known as scab or crust.

Characteristic of Abrasions

1. Grossly or with the aid of hand lens the injury consists of parallel linear injuries which are in line with the direction of the rub or friction causing it;
2. It may exhibit the pattern of the wounding material; and it develops at the precise point of impact of the force, causing it; and it is usually ignored by the attending physician for it does not require medical treatment but it has importance in the medico legal view point.

a. Abrasions caused by ûnger nails may indicate struggle or assault and are usually located in the face, neck, chest, forearms and hands.

b. Abrasions resulting front friction on rough surfaces, either intentional or accidental are located on bony parts of the body and usually associated with contusion and laceration.

c. Nature of the abrasions may infer the damage or pressure nature of the rubbing object and the direction of movement.

Forms of Abrasions

1. *Linear*

An abrasion which appears as a-single line. It may be at straight or curved line. Pinching with the fingernails will produce a linear curved abrasion, while sliding the point of a needle on the skin will produce a straight linear abrasion.

2. Multi-Linear

An abrasion which develops when the skin is rubbed on hard rough object thereby producing several linear marks parallel to one another. This is frequently seen among victims of vehicular accident.

3. Confluent

An abrasion where the linear marks on the skin are almost indistinguishable on account of the severity of the friction and roughness of the object.

4. Multiple

Several abrasions of varying sizes and shapes may be found in different parts of the body.

Types of Abrasions

1. Scratch

This is caused by a sharp-pointed object which slides across the skin, like a pin, thorn or ûngernail. The injury is always parallel to the direction of the slide. The commencement and termination are well deûned and depth depends on the pressure applied. The ûngernails scratch maybe broad at the point of commencement and may terminate with a tailing.

2. Graze

This is usually caused by forcible contact with rough hard object resulting to irregular removal of the kin surface. The nature of injury is dependents upon the degree of roughness of the object and the amount of pressure in the course of the sliding. The course will be indicated by a clean commencement and tags on the end.

3. Impact or Imprint Abrasion

This is a patterned abrasion, stamping abrasion or abrasion a la signature and those whose pattern and location provides objective evidence to show cause, nature of the wounding material and the manner of assault or death.

a. Marked grid of the radiator may be imprinted on the skin.
b. Tire heads marks may be seen in the skin in vehicular accident.
c. Muzzle imprints in the contact fire gunshot wound of entrance; and teeth impression mark in skin bites.

4. Pressure of Friction Abrasion

This is abrasion caused by pressure accompanied by strangulation. The spiral. strands of the rope may be reflected on the skin of the neck.

Differential Diagnosis

1. Dermal Erosion

This is the gradual breakdown or a very shallow ulceration of the skin which involves only the epidermis and heals without scarring.

It may appear in spots and with no previous history of friction or sliding.

2. Marks of Insects and Fishes Bites

The skin injury is irregular with no vital reaction and usually found on angles of the mouth, margins of nose, eyelids and forehead.

3. Excoriation of the Skin by Excreta

This condition is only found among infants and the red skin lesion heals when the cause is removed. There is no apparent history of rubbing trauma on the affected area.

4. Pressure Sore

It is usually found at the back of the region of bony prominence. History of long standing illness bed ridded condition although pressure sore may start as a previous area of abrasion.

Point of Distinction	**Ante-Mortem** Abrasion	**Post-Mortem** Abrasion
Color	Reddish-bronze is appearance due to slight exudation of blood	Yellowish and translucent in appearance.

Location	Any area	Generally occurs overbony prominence, such as elbow, and attributed to rough handling of the cadaver.
Vital Reaction	With intra-vital reaction and may show remains of damaged epithelium	Shows no vital reaction and is characterized by a separation of the epidermis from the complete loss of the former.

b. Incised wound; Cut, Slash or Slice

This is produced by a sharp-edged cutting or sharp-linear edge of the instrument, like a knife, razor, bolo, edge of oyster shell, metal sheet, glass, etc. It may be an impact cut when there is forcible contact of the cutting instrument with the body surface, or slice cut when cutting injury is due to the pressure accompanied with movement of the instrument.

When the wounding instrument is a heavy cutting instrument, like axe, the wound produced is called clipped or shacked wound. The injury is quite severe, and edges may or may not be contused depending on the nature of the sharpness of the instrument used in producing the wounds.

Characteristics of Incised Wounds

1. Edges are clean-out and both extremities are sharp, except in areas where the skin is loose or folded at the time when the injury was inflicted.
2. The wound is straight and may be shelving if inflicted with the wounding instrument applied with an acute angle to the surface of the body involved.
3. Because the blood vessels involved are clean cut profuse hemorrhage is invariably a feature.

4. Gaping is usually present due to retraction of the edges but its presence and degree of retraction depends on the direction of the incised wound with the line of cleavage Langer's Line.
5. If the incised Wound is located in parts of the body covered with clothes, the clothing itself will show clean-cut of the cloth textures and fibers.
6. Usually the Wound is shallow near the extremities and deeper at the middle portion. However, this findings may be modified by the shape of the wounding instrument and the part of the body involved in the application of external stimuli.
7. In the absence of complication and/or when there is no deeper involvement present, healing is relatively fast and the scar may not or may develop colispicuously.
8. Incised wound; caused by broken edges of the glass may be irregular and may appear like a punctured or stab wound. Fragments of the glass may be removed from tile incised wound. Examination with the aid of a magnifying lens is necessary to determine the presence and removal of particles of flakes of glasses in the wound.

Suicidal, Homicidal or Accidental Wounds

1. Suicidal

Located in peculiar parts of the body, like the neck, flexor surfaces of the extremities i.e., elbow, groin, knee, wrist, and accessible to the hand in inflicting the injury. The most common instrument used is the barber's razor blade with an improvised handle.

There are usually superficial tentative cut; hesitation cuts, and the direction varies with the location and the hand; left or right used in inflicting the injuries. The most common site of suicidal incised wound was on the wrist with involvement of the radial artery and the neck.

2. Homicidal

The incised wounds- are deep, multiple and involve both accessible and non-accessible parts of the body to the hands of the victim. Defense and other forms of wounds may be present. Clothing is always involved.

3. Accidental

Multiple incised wound is commonly observed on the passengers and driver of vehicular accidents on account of the broken windshield and glass parts of windows. Stepping on oyster shell, broken glasses, sharp edges of metal sheets are common causes of incised wound on the sole of the foot.

Those associated in the use of kitchen knives in the preparation of food, carpenters and handicraft workers who - use sharp edged instruments are frequent victims of accidental incised wounds.

c. Stab Wound

Stab wound is produced by the penetration of a sharp pointed and sharp edge instrument, like a knife, saber, dagger, and scissors. It may involve the skin or mucous surface. If the sharp edge portion of the wounding instrument is the first to come in contact with the skin, the wound produced is an incised wound, but if the sharp pointed portions first come in contact, then the wound is a stab wound.

As a general rule, like an incised wound, the edges are clean,-cut, regular and distinct. The surface length of a stab wound may reflect the width of the wounding instrument. It may be smaller When the wound is not so deep in as much as it is only caused by the penetration of the tapering portion of the pointed instrument.

It may be made wider if the withdrawal is not on the same direction when it was introduced or the stabbing is accompanied by a slashing movement. In the latter case, the presence of an abrasion from the extremity of the skin is in line with direction of the slashing movement.

The extremities of stab wound may show the nature of the instrument used. A double bladed weapon may cause the production of both extremities sharp. A single bladed instrument may produce as one of its extremities rounded and contused.

This distinction may not be clearly observed if the instrument is quite thin. The direction of the surface defect may be useful in the determination of the possible relative position of the offender and the victim when the wound was inflicted. As to whether the wound is a slit like or gaping depends on the looseness of the skin and the direction of the wound to the line of cleavage - Langer's Line.

The depth may be influence by the size and sharpness of the instrument, area of the body involved, and the degree of force applied. Involvement of the bones may cause clean out fracture on it. A portion of the wounding instrument, usually the tapering part, may remain -in. the body. X-ray examinations may be needed to reveal its location. Hemorrhage is always the most serious consequence of stab would. This is due to the severance of blood vessels or involvement of bloody organs.

Inclusions in Description of a Stab Wound

1. Length of the Skin Defect

The edges must be coaptated before the length is measured. If the abrasion tailing is present in one of the extremities, it must, not be included in the measurement. The length of the tailing must be mentioned separately. The tailing infers direction of withdrawal of the wounding weapon.

2. Condition of Extremities

A sharp extremity may infer the sharpness of the edge of the instrument used. If both extremities are sharp, it may be inferred that a double bladed weapon was used.

3. Condition of the Edges

If the injury is due to stabbing act, the edges are regular and clean cut. However, if the wound is caused by several stabbing acts, i.e., series of thrust and withdrawal, the edges may be serrated, or zigzag in appearance.

4. Linear Direction of Surface Wound

It may be running vertically, horizontally, or upward medially or laterally.

5. Location of the Stab Wound

Aside from mentioning the region of body where the wound is located, its exact measurement to some anatomical landmarks must be stated.

6. Direction of Penetration

This must be tri-dimensional, backwards or forwards, upwards or downwards, and medially or laterally.

7. Depth of Penetration

8. Tissue and Organs Involved

1. Evidence showing that the stab wound is suicidal:

a. It is located over the vital parts of the body.

b. It is usually solitary. If multiple, they are located on one part of the body.

c. If located on covered parts of the body the clothing re not involved.

d. The stab Wound is accessible to the hand of the victim.

e. The hand of the victim is sin eared with blood.

f. The wounding weapon is firmly grasped -by the hand of the victim-cadaveric spasm.

g. If stabbing is accompanied with slashing movement, the wound tailing abrasion is seen towards the hand inflicting the injury.

h. A suicide note may be present.

i. There is presence of a motive for self-destruction.

j. No disturbance in the death scene, wounding instrument is found near the victim.

2. Evidence showing that the stab wound is homicidal:

a. Injuries other than stab Wound may be present, stab: wound may be located in any part of the body, and usually there are more than one stab wound.

b. There is a motive for the stabbing. If without motive the offender must be insane or under the influence of drugs, and there is disturbance in the crime scene.

3. Medical Evidences Showing Intent of the Offender to Kill the Victim

a. There are more than one stab wounds, and stab wounds are deep, and the stab wound are located in different parts of the body or on parts of the body Where vital organs are located.

b. Stab wound with serrated or zigzag borders infers alternative thrust and withdrawal of the wounding weapon to increase internal damages.

c. Irregular or stellate shape skin defects may be due to changing direction of the weapon with portion of the instrument at the level of the skin as the lever. In this way a greater area of involvement internally will be realized.

Different measurement of the stab wounds may possibly be produced by one weapon if it is tapering towards the sharp point. Withdrawal of the instrument not on the ' same direction as when it was introduced may increase the length of the skin defect.

A sharpened three cornered object, when used as a stabbing weapon will produce three cornered extremities, skin defect. The most common immediate cause of death is hemorrhage particularly when located in the chest or abdomen.

Accidental stab wounds are quite rare and are usually caused by falling against a projecting sharp object like broken pieces of glass or flattened and pointed iron bars.

d. Punctured Wound

Punctured wound is the result of a thrust of a sharp pointed instrument. The external injury is quite small but the depth is to a certain degree. It is commonly produced by an ice-pick, needle, nail, spear, pointed stick, thorn, fang of animal and hook.

The nature of the external injury depends on the sharpness and shape of the end of the wounding instrument. Contusion of the edges may be present if the end is not so sharp. The opening maybe round, elliptical, diamond-shape or cruciate.

An accurate cross section nature of the wounding object may be well appreciated when there is involvement of flat hard parts of the body especially the skull. External hemorrhage is quite limited although internal injuries may be severe. However direct involvement of blood vessels and bloody organs may cause fatal consequences unless appropriate medical intervention is applied.

The site of the external wound can be easily sealed by the dried blood, vessels and bloody organs clotted blood so that introduction of pathogenic microorganism which does not require the presence of air in its growth multiplication may find the place favorable and may produce fatal consequences. Punctured wound is usually accidental but in rare instances it may be homicidal or suicidal.

Characteristics of Punctured Wounds

1. The opening on the skin is very small and may become unnoticeable because of clotted blood and elasticity of the skin. The wound is much deeper than it is wide.
2. External hemorrhage is limited although internally it may be severe.
3. Sealing of the external opening will be favorable for the growth and multiplication of anaerobic microorganism such as like bacillus tetani.

Evidence to Show it is Homicidal

1. It is multiple and usually located in the different parts of the body. It may however be found in certain areas of the body.
2. The wound are deep, there are defense wounds on the victim, and there is disturbance in the crime scene sign of struggle or presence of violence.

Proof to Show it is Suicidal

1. Located in areas of the body where the vital organs are located, and usually singular but may be multiple and located in one area of 'the body'.
2. Parts of the body involved is accessible to the hand of the victim, and clothing usually is not involved.
3. 'Wounding is made by the weapon while the victim is in sitting or standing position. There is bleeding towards the lower part of body or clothing.
4. No disturbance of the crime scene, presence of suicide note, and wounding instrument found near the body of the victim.

Caused by Poisonous Instrument

1. Poison dart; cyanide or nicotine, fish spines, and dog bites with hydrophobia virus.
2. Injection of Air and Poison as a way of euthanasia. i.e., lacerated wound, tear, rupture, stretch.

Lacerated wound is a tear of the skin and the underlying tissues due to forcible contact with blunt instrument. It may be produced by a hit with a piece of wood, iron bar, first blow, stone, butt of firearm, or other objects without sharp objects. If the force applied to a tissue is greater than its cohesive force and elasticity, the tissue tears and a laceration is produced.

Since the skin is composed of several types of tissues, namely: epidermis, connective tissue, fat, blood vessels, nerves, glandular cells, etc. each having its own breaking point, the laceration will be irregular and having strands of tissues bridging. The rupture of continuity may only extend deeper to the stronger layer like that of the galea aponeuritica in case of scalp injury.

Characteristics of Lacerated Wounds

1. The shape and size of the injury do not correspond of the wounding instrument.
2. The tear on the skin is rugged with extremities irregular and ill-defined.
3. The injury developed is at the site where the blunt force is applied.
4. The borders of the wound are contused and swollen.
5. It is usually developed on the areas of the body where the bone is superficially located. Like the scalp, face, legs; and foot, etc.,
6. Examination with the aid of the hand lens show bridging tissue joining the edges and hair bulbs intact.
7. Bleeding is not extensive because the blood vessels are severed evenly and healing process is delayed and has more tendency to develop scar.

Classifications of Lacerated Wound

1. Splitting caused by crushing of the skin between two hard objects.

This is best seen in laceration of the scalp caused by a hit of a blunt instrument, cut eyebrow of boxer and laceration of the chin of motorcyclist.

2. *Overstretching of the Skin*

When pressure is applied on one side of the bone, the skin over the area will be stretched up to breaking point to cause laceration and exposure of the fractured bones. In avulsion, the edge of the remaining tissue is that of laceration.

3. *Grinding Compression*

The weight and the grinding movement may cause separation of the skin with the underlying tissue.

4. *Tearing*

This may be produced by a semi-sharp instrument which causes irregular edges on the wound, like hatchet and choppers. Laceration wounds may involve deeper tissues like laceration of the muscles and fracture of bones depending upon the degree of force applied in causing it. It may be homicidal or accidental but rarely, it is suicidal. An insane person may hit his head on a concrete Wall but when loss of consciousness develop she will not be able to continue further his act of self-destruction.

Incised Wound vs. Lacerated Wound

Incised Wound	Lacerated Wound
Edges are clean-cut, regular and well defined.	Edges are roughly cut, irregular and ill-defined.
There is no swelling or contusion around the incised lacerated wound.	There is swelling and contusion around the wound.
Extremities of the wound are sharp or may be round or contused.	Extremities of the wound are ill-defined and irregular.

Examination by means of magnifying lens shows that the hair is cut.	Examination with a magnifying lens shows that hair bulbs are presented.
Healing is faster:	Healing is
Scar is linear or spindle types.	delayed. Scar is
It is caused by sharp edge instrument.	irregular

Gaping Wound

It is the separation of the edges especially in deep. Would may be due to the following:

1. Mechanical Stretching

The presence of a mechanical device on the edges to –prevent coaptation will cause separation. The presence of a canula in tracheostomy, drain rubber or gauze in an incise abscess, or a retractor during operation are examples of this type of gaping.

2. Loss of Tissue

Separation of the edges of a wound may be on account of loss of tissue bridging them, the loss of the body tissue maybe due to the following.

a. Destruction by pressure, infection, cell lysis, burning or chemical. reaction, and avulsion or physical or mechanical; stretching resulting to separation of a portion of the tissue.
b. Trimming of the edges or debridment of the skin which come in contact with the bullet at the gunshot wound-of entrance and the removal of the 'necrotic material in an infected wound may cause separation of the edges.

3. Retraction of the Edges

Underneath the skin are dense networks of fibrous and elastic connective tissue fibers running on the same direction and forming a pattern more of) less present in persons. This pattern of fiber arrangement is called cleavage direction or lines of cleavage of the skin and their linear representation on the skin is called Langers Line, These lines of cleavage are different in different parts of the body.

If an incised wound or stab wound was inflicted wherein the long axis of the wound is parallel or on the same directions as the cleavage line of the part of the body involved, the wound will appear narrow or slit-like because the edges of the wound will not be subjected to the lateral pull of the severed connective tissue fibers. If the long axis of the wound is perpendicular to or with an angle with the lines of cleavage, the tendency of the borders of the wound is to separate on account of the retraction of the severed fibers.

Fatal Effects of Wounds

The following are the fatal effects of wounds:

l. Wound may be Directly Fatal by Reason of:

a. Hemorrhage

An incised wound at the lateral aspect of the neck involving the carotid artery without surgical intervention is fatal due to hemorrhage. While wounds in some areas of the body where big blood vessels are not present and the reaction of tissue are strong, death will not be a direct result due to hemorrhage ill the absence of complication that may set it.

b. Mechanical Injuries on the Vital Organs

A blow on the head may not necessarily produced external lesions, but may produce severe meningeal hemorrhage producing compression of the brain. A punctured wound of the heart, even though how small, may produce sudden death on account of the tamponade of the heart.

2. Wound may be Indirectly Fatal by Reason of:

a. Secondary Hemorrhage Following Sepsis

A wound because of its nature and location is not capable of producing severe hemorrhage, but on account of infection that set in, deeper tissues are involved including big blood vessels thereby producing severe hemorrhage.

b. Specific Infection

Pathogenic microorganisms may develop and multiply in the wound causing septicemia, bacteremia, or toxemia. Tetanus, gas gangrene infections are common in open wounds.

c. Scarring Effect

Chronic gonorrhea infection may cause stricture of the uretha. Stricture of the esophagus may follow ingestion of irritant poison. Keloid formation in burns may not only cause deformity but disturbance of the normal respiration of locomotion.

Complications of Trauma or Injury

Hereunder are complications of brought about by trauma or injury caused by external stimuli:

1. Shock

Shock is the disturbance of fluid balance resulting to peripheral deficiency which is manifested by the decreased volume of blood, reduced volume of flow, hemo concentration and renal deficiency. It is clinically characterized by severe depression of the brain and the central nervous system.

There are three major factors that operate in the production of shock and all are likely to be associated together as the condition develops, as follows: extensive injury to the receptive nervous system; anoxemia reduction of the effective volume of oxygen carrying capacity of the blood; and endothelial damage, which thus increases the capillary permeability.

Kinds of Shock

a. Primary Shock

This is caused by immediate nerve impulse set up at the injured area which is conveyed to the central nervous system. The impulse may also whelm the vital centers in the medulla thereby shock develops within a short time due to vasomotor collapse. If the reaction is not intense, the patient may live longer or may recover completely from the effect of shock.

b. Delayed or Secondary Shock

Patient shows signs of general collapse which develop sometime after the infliction of injury. It is characterized by a low blood pressure, subnormal temperature, cold clammy perspiration. The shock may be severe to produce death or the patient may recover completely from its effect.

2. Hemorrhage

Hemorrhage is the extravasations or loss of blood from the circulation brought about by wounds in the cardio-vascular system. The degree and nature of hemorrhage depends upon the size, kind and location of the blood vessel cut, and types of the weapon used in producing the physical injury.

Kinds of Hemorrhage

Primary Hemorrhage

It is the bleeding which occurs immediately after the traumatic injury of the blood vessel.

Secondary Hemorrhage

This occurs not immediately after the infliction of the injury but Sometime thereafter on or near the injured area.

3. Infection

Infection is the appearance, growth and development of micro-organism at the site of injury.

How Injury or Trauma Acquires Infections

a. From the instrument or substance which produces the physical injury.
b. From the organs involved in the trauma applied. A bullet wound may involve the intestine and causes its contents to spill out in the peritoneal cavity causing peritonitis.
c. As indirect effect of the injury which creates a local area of diminished resistance causing the invasion and multiplication of microorganism.
d. Injury may depress the general vitality, especially among the aged and the young children and makes the patient succumb

to terminal disease, and deliberate introduction of microorganisms at the site of the physical injury.

4. Embolism

This is a condition in which foreign matters are introduced in the blood stream causing sudden block to the blood flow in the finer arterioles and capillaries.

Most Common Emboli in the Blood Stream

Fat embolus, that is by injection of oily substance into direction of the blood flow, and by injury of the adipose tissue which forces fat into the circulation. Air embolism, that is due to gaping incised wound of the jugular vein, and injection of soapsuds or air into pregnant uterus for the purpose of tubal insuflation or criminal abortion.

Through the injection of air into the urinary bladder for purposes of radiological study, insuflation of other non-potent tubes or the hollow organs of the body, and injection of air under pressure into the nasal sinus after therapeutic lavage.

Describing the Physical Injuries

Because some injuries may be either accidental or inflicted, diagnosing abuse is not as simple as diagnosing, for example, appendicitis. Effective differential diagnosis, the process of distinguishing abusive from accidental injuries, relies upon a clinician's ability to make the connection between the injuries described by the victims.

For purposes of presenting the corpus delicti during trial of the case, the trauma suffered by the victim must be described by the medico-legal officer as serious, less serious and slightly serious physical injuries, indicating the said findings in the medical certificate issued relatively with the case, and serve as basis on the part of the investigator in filing the necessary case against the suspect to the proper court.

7

Investigation of Wounds

The following rules must always be observed by the physician in the examination of wounds, i.e., all injuries must be described, however small for it may be important later, the description of the wounds must be comprehensive, and if possible a sketch or photograph must be taken, and the examination must not be influenced by any other information obtained from other in making a report or conclusion.

Outline of Investigation

Hereunder is the outline of the investigation of wounds:

1. General Investigation of the-Surroundings

a. Examination of the place where the crime was committed

1. Examination of the clothing, stains, cuts, hairs and other foreign bodies that can be found in the scene of the crime.
2. Investigation of those persons who may be the witnesses to the incident or those who could give light to the case.
3. Examination of the wounding instrument.
4. Photograph, sketching, or accurate description of the scene of the crime for purposes of preservation.

b. Examination of the Wounded Body

1. Examinations that are applicable to the living and dead body.
2. Age of the wound from the degree of healing.
3. Determination of the weapon used in the commission of the offense.

4. Reasons for the multiplicity of wounds in cases where there are more than one wound.
5. Determination whether the injury is accidental, suicidal or homicidal.

c. Examinations that is applicable only to the living

1. Determination whether the injury is dangerous to life.
2. Determination whether the injury will produce permanent deformity.
3. Determination whether the wound was produced by is shock or not.
4. Determination whether the injury will produce complication.

d. Examinations that is applicable to the dead victim

1. Determination whether the wound is ante-mortem or post-mortem.
2. Determination whether the wound is mortal or not.
3. Determination whether the death is accelerated by a disease or some abnormal developments which are present at the time of the infliction of wound.
4. Determination whether the wound was caused by accident, suicide or homicide.

2. Examination of the Wound

The following must be included in the examination of the wound. The report made in connection with such examination must also include in detail the following items:

a. Character of the Wound

The description must first state the type of wound, e.g., abrasion, contusion, hematoma, incised, lacerated, stab wound, etc. It must include the size, shape, nature of the edges, extremities and other characteristic marks. The presence of contusion collar in case of gunshot wound of entrance, scab formation in abrasion and other open wounds, infection, surgical intervention, etc., must also be stated.

b. Location of the Wound

The region of the body where the wound is situated must be stated.

It is advisable to measure the distance of the wound from some fixed point of the body prominence to facilitate reconstruction. This is important in determining the trajectory or course of the wounding weapon inside the body.

c. Depth of the Wound

The determination of the exact depth of the wound must not be attempted in a living subjects if in so doing it will prejudice the health or life. Depth is measurable is the outer wound and the inner end is fixed. No attempt must be made in measuring the stabbed wound of the abdomen because of the mot/ability of the abdominal wall.

d. Condition of the Surroundings

The area surrounding the wound must be examined. In gunshot wound near or contact fire will produce burning or tattooing of the surrounding skin. In suicidal wound, there may be superficial tentative cuts, hesitation cuts. Lacerated wound may show contusion of the neighboring skin.

e. Extent of the Wound

Extensive injury may show marked degree of force applied in the production of the wound. In homicidal cut-throat cases, it is generally deeper than in cases of suicide. Homicidal wounds are extensive and numerous.

f. Direction of the Wound

The direction of the wound is material in the determination of the relative position of the victim and the offender when such wound has been inflicted. The direction of the incised wound of the anterior aspects of the neck may differentiate whether it is homicidal or suicidal.

g. Number of Wounds

Several wounds found in different parts of the body are generally indicative of murder or homicide.

h. Conditions of the Locality

Study the degree of hemorrhage, evidence of struggle, information as to the position of the body, presence of letter or suicide note, and condition of the weapon.

Wounds Inflicted During Life or Death?

In the determination whether the wounds were inflicted during life or after death, the following factors must be taken into consideration in the conduct of examination:

1. Hemorrhage

As a general rule, hemorrhage is more profuse when the wound was inflicted during the lifetime of the victim. In wounds inflicted after death, the amount of bleeding is comparatively less if at all bleeding occurred. This is due to the loss of tone of the blood vessels, the absence of heart action and post-mortem clotting of blood inside the blood vessels. Violence inflicted on a living body may not show the formation of a bruise until after death.

2. Signs of Inflammation

There may be swelling of the area surrounding the wound, effusion of lymph or pus and adhesion of the edges. Other vital reactions are present whenever the wound was inflicted during life, although it may be less pronounced when resistance of the victim is markedly weakened. The vital reaction may also indicate the time of infliction of the wound. Post-mortem wounds do not show any manifesting signs of vital reactions.

3. Signs of Repair

Fibrin formation, growth of epithelium, scab or scar formations conclusively show that the wound was inflicted during life. But the absence of signs of repair does not show that injury was inflicted after death. The tissue may not have been given ample time to repair itself before death took place.

4. Retraction of the Edges of the Wound

Owing to the vital reactions of the skin and contractility of the muscular fibers, the edge of the wound inflicted during life retracts and cause gaping. On the other hand, in the case of the wound inflicted after death, the edges do not gape are closely approximately to each other because the skin and the muscles have lost their contractility.

Ante-Mortem vs. Post-Mortem Wounds:

Ante-Mortem	Post-Mortem
Hemorrhage more or less copious. Marks of spouting of blood form arteries. Clotted blood.	Hemorrhage slight or none at all and always venous. No spotting of blood. Blood is not clotted, if all is a soft clot.
Deep staining of the edges and cellular tissues, which are not removed by washing.	The edges of the cellular tissues are not deeply stained. The staining can be removed by washing.
The edges gape owing to the reaction of the skin and muscle fibers.	The edges do not gape, but are closely approximated to each other, unless the wound is caused within one or two hours after death.
Inflammation and reparative process.	No inflammation of reparative process.

Homicidal vs. Suicidal vs. Accidental Wounds;

a. External signs and circumstances related to the position and attitude of the body when found.

b. Location of the weapon or the manner in which it was held.

c. The motive underlying the commission of the crime and the like.

d. The personal character of the deceased.

e. The possibility for the offender to have purposely changed the truth of the condition.

f. As to the Nature of the Wound Inflicted

g. Abrasions

Extensive abrasions on the body are always suggestive of accidental death due to traffic accident. In suicidal death, abrasions are rarely observed. In case of murder, abrasions are not common except when the body is dragged on the ground. In homicide, abrasion may commonly be observed, especially when the victim offered some degree of resistance to the attacker.

2. Contusion

Contusion is rarely observed in suicidal death, except when the suicide act was done by jumping from a height. A person contemplating to commit suicide will not choose a blunt instrument.

Contusion in accidental death may also be found in any portion of the body. It is often due to a fall and due to a forcible contact with some hard objects.

3. Incised Wounds

Incised wounds are commonly observed in suicide and homicide. The depth, location and other surroundings circumstances will differentiate one from the other. Accidental cuts are frequent everyday occurrences, but rarely as a cause of death.

4. Other Information;

a. Signs of Struggle

Absence of signs of struggle is more in suicide, accident or murder. Contusion or abrasion may indicate trauma due to fist, finger or feet of the assailant. Presence of hair or portion of the skin on the nails of the assailant or deceased may be a clue in the determination whether death is suicidal, homicidal or accidental.

b. Number and Direction of Wounds

Multiple wounds in concealed portions of the body are generally indicative of homicide. Single wound located in a position that the deceased could have been conveniently inflicted is usually indicative of suicidal wound.

c. Direction of the Wound

This is important in the case of cut-throat. The direction wound is generally transverse in case of homicide while it is oblique in case of suicide.

d. Nature and Extent of the Wound

Homicidal wounds may be brought about by any wound instrument. Suicidal wounds are frequent due to sharp instruments. Accidental physical injuries may be of any kind.

e. State of the Clothing

There is usually no change in the condition of the clothing in suicide càse. In homicidal death, on account of the struggle which took place before death, the clothing of the victim is in a disorderly fashion.

Length of Survival of the Victim

In the approximation of the length of survival of the victim after receipt of the physical injury, the following factors must be taken into considerations, to wit:

1. Changes in Body in Relation to Time of Death

The length of time in the survival of the victim may be approximated from the systematic changes in the body. The degree of wasting, anemia, condition of the face and bed sore formation may be a basic as to how long a person survived.

2. Age of the Blood Stain

The age of the blood stain may be determined from the physical color changes of the skin, although it is not reliable. Although there are some basis for such method, it must not be relied upon because the physical changes of the blood is modified by several external factors.

3. Degree of Healing

The injured portion of the body undergoes certain chemical and physical changes as a normal course of repair. The capillaries are dilated and edema develops at once. This is followed by the migration of the white cells from the capillaries to the damage area.

Fibroblast begin to proliferate later with the formation of the granulation tissues. Sings of repair of the wound appear in less than a day after the infliction of injury. By the degree of granulation tissue formation and other reparative changes, the age -of the wound may be estimated.

4. Testimony of Witness When Wound was Inflicted

The actual witness may testify in courts as to exact time the wound was inflicted by the offender. In this case, medical evidence as to the duration of survival is merely corroborative.

Possible Instrument Used by Assailant

The determination of the wounding instrument may be made from the nature of the wound found in the body of the victim:

1. Contusion-produced by blunt object or instrument, usually; by hitting the victim.
2. Incised wound-produced by sharp-edged instrument inflicted by hitting.
3. Lacerated wound-produced by blunt instrument.
4. Puncture wound-produced by sharp-pointed instrument.
5. Abrasion, body surface is rubbed on a rough hind surface.
6. Gunshot wound the diameter of the wound of entrance may approximate the caliber of the wounding fire arm;

Which Injuries Sustained Caused Death?

If there are several offenders who conspired with one another in the commission of the offense, it is not necessary to determine who among them gave the fatal blow. In the crime of conspiracy, the act of one is the act of all. But if there is no conspiracy in the commission of the offense it is necessary to determine who among the offenders gave the fatal injury to the victim, because they are only responsible for their individual acts.

In a case wherein the victim is a recipient of multiple injuries, the determination as to which of the injuries causes death is dependent on the testimony of the physician. This can be ascertained by examining individually the wounds and note which of them are involved in the injury to some vital organs or large vessels, or led to secondary results causing death.

When two or more wound involved the vital organs, it is difficult to ascertain which among them caused the death. It is important to determine the degree of the damage of each of the wound cause on the vital organ.

Which Wound was Inflicted First?

Where there are several. wounds presents on the body of the victim, it is important to determine which of them was inflicted first because it may be necessary for the qualification of the offense committed. If the first wound was inflicted in a treacherous way that the victim after receipt is incapable of defense then murder is committed, but if the fatal wound was inflicted last, it is possible that the crime committed is only homicide.

In the determination as to which of the wounds present was inflicted first, the following factors must be taken into consideration:

1. Relative position of the assailant and the victim when the first injury was inflicted on the latter.
2. Trajectory of course of the wound inside the body of the victim.
3. Organs involved and the degree of injury sustained by the victim.
4. Testimony of witness.
5. Presence of defense wounds on the victim. If the victim tried to make a defensive act during the initial attack, then the defense wounds must have been inflicted first.

Surgical Intervention Before Death

If the death of the victim followed a surgical or-medical intervention, the offender will still be held responsible for -the death-of the victim it can be proven that death was inevitable and that even -Without the operation, death is normal and direct consequences of the injuries sustained unto the person of the deceased.

It must be competent and that in spite his exercise of care and diligence, still death was the final outcome. A person committing a felony shall be responsible for whatever will be the outcome of his felonious act.

The wound inflicted by him must be the direct and proximate cause of the death of the victim.

On the other hand, if the victim merely received minor wounds but death resulted on account of the gross incompetence or negligence of the physician, then the offender cannot be held responsible" for the death. The offender can only be made responsible for the physical "injuries inflicted on the victim and the physician must be made to answer for the death of the victim.

Negligence on the Death of Person

If death occurred from complications arising from a simple. Injury owing to the negligence of the injured person in its proper care and treatment; the offender is still held responsible for the death. A person is not bound to submit himself to medical treatment for the injuries received during the assault.

The fact that the victim would have lived had he received appropriate medical attention is immaterial. Hence the refusal of the deceased to be operated does not relieve the offender of the criminal liability for his death. But, it could be proven-that the negligence of the victim is deliberate and that his intention is really the cause of death on himself, then the offender -cannot be held responsible for the death, but only for the physical injuries he inflicted.

Power of Volitional Act of the Victim

Sometimes it is necessary to determine whether a victim of a fatal wound is still capable of speaking, walking or performing any other volitional acts. A dying declaration may be presented by the prosecutor mentioning the accused as the assailant, the offender may allege that the physical injuries inflicted by him while the victim was or that the victim inside his house and that he walked for some; distance where he fell, or that the victim after the fatal injury made an attempt to inflicted injuries to the accused which justified that latter to give another fatal blow.

The determination of the victims capacity to perform volitional acts rests upon the medical witness. As a general rule, sever injury of the brain and the cranial box usually produces unconsciousness, but after a while, the victim may be capable of performing volitional acts. The power to perform volitional acts is dependent upon the area of the brain involved.

Wounds of the big blood vessels, like the carotid, jugular; or even the aorta. Do not prevent a person from exercising voluntary acts or even from running a certain distance. Penetrating wound of the heart is often considered to be instantaneously fatal but experience show that the victim may still be capable of locomotion. Rupture of the organ is not always followed by death. The victim has for sometimes still retains the capacity to move and speak.

Extreme caution must be exercised by the physician in express his opinion to the limitation of powers possessed by the injured person to perform acts of volition, locomotion, or speech subsequent to receipt of extensive or fatal injury or wound.

Relative Position of the Victim and Assailant

In the determination of the relative position of the victim and the assailant, the following points must be considered by the physician:

1. Location of the wound in the body of the victim.
2. Direction of the wound.
3. Nature of the instrument used in inflicting the injury.
4. Testimony of witnesses.

Extrinsic Evidences in Wounds

The following are the extrinsic evidences in wounds:

1. Evidence from the Wounding Weapon a. Position of the Weapon

The location and position of the weapon at the scene of the crime may afford strong evidence in the court. As a rule, in cases of accidental or suicidal death, the wounding weapon is found near the body of the victim; but it is not uncommon to find the victim at some distance front the weapon when the victim is capable of walking. If the wounding instrument is firmly grasped by the victim, it is a strong presumption that it is suicidal case.

b. Blood of Weapon

The weapon responsible for the production of wound may be stained with blood. In some instances, the wounding weapon does not show blood stains because of the rapidity of the blow and compression of the blood vessels. Even if the weapon is stained with blood, it may be wiped out by the clothing in the process of withdrawal.

c. Hair and Other Substance on Weapon

Hair or fibers of cotton, silk, linen another fabrics may be found adhering on the weapon. It must be preserved and submitted for comparison with the clothing or hair found at the site of the injury on the victim body.

2. Evidences in the Clothing of the Victim

Injuries inflicted on the covered portions of the body may also show injury on the covered apparel. In gunshot Wound, the hole in the clothing may be a factor in the determination of the site of the wound entrance. Occasionally, two or more tears or holes are produced on the dress by a single wound. This can be explained by the presence of folds on the clothing. In gunshot Wound, determination of the presence of gunpowder at the hole of entrance may show distance. The prominence of clean cut tear in the clothing shows that a sharp- edged instrument was used. The presence of severe tearing of the clothing shows struggle. The degree of soaking of the clothing with blood may depict the degree of hemorrhage.

3. Evidence from the Examination of the Assailant

The clothing of the assailant may be stained with blood from the victim. Tear may be present on account of the struggle which existed at the time of the commission of the offense. The ûngernails may show foreign substance coming from the body of the victim. The offender may also slow -to a certain degree marks of violence. Paraffin test of the assailant's hands may be useful to determine whether he fired the gun in case of shooting. Determination of the degree of intoxication, mental condition, physical power, etc. of the offender may be necessary in the solution of crime.

4. Evidence Derived from the Scene of the Crime

The condition of the surrounding objects, the amount of hemorrhage, the presence of identifying articles belonging to the victim or assailant, the wounding instrument, all these must be observed or collected by the investigator.

8

Medico Legal Aspects of Sex Crimes

In general, laws prescribe acts which are considered either sexual abuse, or behavior that societies consider to be inappropriate and against the social norms. In addition, certain categories of activity may be considered crimes even if freely consented to. Sex laws vary from place to place, and over time. Sexual acts W- which are prohibited by law in a jurisdiction, are also called sex crimes.

Definition of Virginity

Virginity is a condition of a female who has not experienced sexual intercourse and whose genital organs have not been altered by carnal connection. A woman is virtuous female body is pure and if she has never had any sexual intercourse with another, though her mind and heart is impure.

A woman is presumed to be a virgin when unmarried and of good reputation. Unlike the term premarital sex, which can refer to more than one occasion of sexual activity and can be judgment neutral, the concept of virginity usually. involves moral or religious issues and can have consequences in terms of social status and in interpersonal relationships.

Kinds of Virginity

Hereunder are the different kinds of virginity that are considered an important considerations with regards medico-legal aspects of rape and other sexual offenses:

1. Moral Virginity

This is the state of not knowing the nature of sexual life and not having experienced sexual relation. Moral virginity applies to children below the age of puberty and whose sex organs and secondary sex characters are not yet developed.

2. Physical Virginity

A condition whereby a woman conscious of the nature of the sexual life but has not experienced sexual intercourse. The term applies to women who have reached sexual maturity but have not experienced sexual intercourse. During medico-legal examinations it is really hard to deduce a conclusive and accurate medical finding to show that a woman is physically virgin.

Reliance is given to the absence of laceration of the hymen, but woman might have had previous sexual intercourse and yet the hymen was un-ruptured, while other might not have experienced of sexual relations but have laceration of the hymen. If the findings show absence of laceration of the hymen, distinction should be drawn between true and false physical virginity.

a. True Physical Virginity

It is a condition. wherein the hymen of the female under examination is intact with the edges distinct and regular and the opening are small to barely admit the tip of the smaller finger of the examiner even if the thighs are separated.

b. False Physical Virginity

A condition wherein the hymen is un-ruptured but the orifice is wide and elastic to admit two or more fingers of the examiner with lesser degree of resistance. The hymen may be relaxed and distensible and may have previous sexual relation, In this particular instance the physician not be able to make convincing conclusion that the subject of the medico- legal examination is virgin.

3. Demi Virginity

This term refers to a condition of a woman who permits any form of sexual liberties as long as they abstain from rupturing their hymen by sexual act. The woman may be embraced; kissed, may allow her breast to be fondled, her private parts to be held and other lascivious acts. The woman allows sexual intercourse but only inter-femora or even inter-labia but not to the extent of rupturing the hymen.

4. Virgo Intacta

Literally the term refers to a truly virgin woman; that there are no structural changes in her organ to infer previous sexual intercourse and that she is virtuous woman. In as much as there are no conclusive evidences to prove the existence of such condition, liberal authorities extend the connotation of the term to include women who have had previous sexual act or eventually but had not given birth.

Determination of the Conditions of Virginity

Hereunder are parts of the female body to be considered in the determination of the conditions of virginity.

1. Breasts

The breasts mammary glands, are functionally related to the reproductive system since they secrete milk for nourishment of the young child. At their inner structures are 15 to 20 lobes of glandular tissues supported by connective tissue framework with variable amount of adipose tissue. On the ventral surface of each breast is a cylindrical projection called nipple with perforations which are the openings of the ducts draining the milk glands.

The nipple is surrounded by a pigmented area called areola which becomes dark brown during pregnancy. The size, consistency and shape of the female adult breast varied with age, degree of physical development, stage in the menstrual cycle, pregnancy, nutrition and hormonal factors. A fully developed breast may be classified according to shape:

a. Hemispherical Breast

The breast is like a hemisphere. The contour lines are not straight but form part of a circle or half of a sphere.

b. Conical Breast

The breast has the shape similar to a cone. The outline consists-of two converging lines which meet at the region of the nipple.

c. Infantile or Flat Breast

The breast is only slightly elevated from the chest without distinct boundary and showing no definite shape.

d. Pendulous Breast

The skin of the breast is loose making it capable of swinging in any direction. This is commonly observed among parturient breast-feeding mothers. A pendulous breast may be:

1. Hemispherical pendulous breast - it has the shape of a hemisphere but with loose skin.
2. Conical pendulous breast - it has the shape of a cone and is capable of swinging sidewise.

The condition of the breast is not a reliable evidence to determine virginity. The size, shape and consistency of the breast may be hormonal or hereditary. The advent of artificial feeding makes it possible for parturient women to preserve the condition of the breast. During any sexual related activities, breast size increases, venous patterns "across the breasts become more visible, and nipples harden. Compared to other primates, human breasts are proportionately large throughout adult life the females lives.

2. Vaginal Canal

As a general rule, the vaginal canal of a virgin is tight and the rugosities are sharp and prominent. Insertion of a finger or instrument may show certain degree of resistance. The wall of the vagina is composed of smooth muscle and fibro-elastic connective tissue so that its tightness and degree of resistance on insertion of a finger or an instrument depends on the integrity of its wall, as well as on the potency of its lubricating secretion.

The sharpness of the vaginal wall's rugosities may be diminished by insertion of foreign bodies, passage of clotted blood, self-manipulation, etc. and not by sexual intercourse. The canal may be inherently lax and rugosities not prominent since birth.

3. Labia Majora and Labia Minora

The labia majora is firm, elastic and plump and its medial borders are usually in close contact with each other so as to cover the labia minora and the clitoris. The labia minora is soft, pinkish in close contact with one another, and its vestibule is narrow. Entry of the male organ may cause the labia to gape due to stretching of their borders. The condition of both labia is nota reliable basis in determining virginity.

A woman may be a Virgin but with gaping labia, while others might have had previous delivery but the labia are still coaptated. The condition of the labia is much more related to the general physical condition of the woman rather than the absence or the presence of previous sexual inter course A stout Woman usually can preserve the plump, coaptated and firm labia while skinny have gaping labia.

4. Fourchette

The fourchette present V-shape appearances as the two labias unite posteriorly. After severe distention, the sharpness of the acute angle may become rounded with retraction of the edges; The rounding of the fourchette and the retraction of the edges can be a consequence of so many causes. Stretching apart of the thighs, instrumentation, horse or bicycle riding may produce the condition other than sexual intercourse.

5. Hymen

Physicians give much attention in the examination of the hymen in the determination of virginity.

Classification of Hymen

a. As to shape and size of opening:

1. Annular or circular — the opening is oval or circular located at the center of the hymen. There may be indentation of the borders.
2. Infantile F the opening is small; usually linear, fleshy and resistant.

3. Semilunar or cresentric - the concavity may be facing either side or upwards or downwards. The tapering ends of the crescent may be the frequent site of laceration.
4. Linear - the opening is slit-like and usually running vertically.
5. Crib-form - the hymen presents several openings instead of a single one. In several instances the openings are quite small and will require the use of a hand lens to make them visible.
6. Stellate - hymenal opening is like a star.
7. Septate - there are two openings which may be of equal or different sizes separated by a bridge of hymenal tissue. After a sexual act there may be a complete rupture of the bridging tissue or marked distention of one to make the other opening almost visible.
8. Fimbriated - the border of the opening shows small irregular protrusion towards the opening. In some instances the fimbriation may be bold enough that the examiner may mistake it to be stiperûcial lacerations.
9. Imperforate - there is no opening on the hymen. When a woman starts to menstruate, surgery may be necessary to open the hymen to allow the free passage of menstrual blood.

b. As to structure and consistency?

1. Firm and with strong connective tissue plenty of blood vessels this type has more tendencies to lacerate during the first sexual act and the laceration may produce relatively more hemorrhage.
2. Thick yielding hymen with scarce blood vessels the hymen is distensible, easily penetrated and when lacerated will cause less bleeding.
3. Membranous hymen - hymen is parchment like, may be transparent and may lacerate without pain or appreciable bleeding.

c. As to number of opening

1. Single Orifiçe - having one opening;
2. Septate - having two openings.

3.' Multiple - having several openings.

4. Imperforate - without orifice.

Virginity is Not Synonymous with Chastity

A woman may resort to many forms of homosexual as well as heterosexual-practices without -losing her virginity, yet she may be unchaste. A woman may have a ruptured hymen and other signs of loss of physical virginity, yet she is chaste. She may resort to masturbation with rupture of the hymen and dilation of the vaginal canal, and causing it to appear that she has had -several sexual intercourses, yet she may still be a virgin.

Defloration Defined

Defloration is the laceration or rupture of the hymen a result of sexual intercourse. All other laceration of the hymen which is not caused by sexual act is not considered as defloration.

Examining Female Genitalia to Determine Virginity

Following are parts of the female genitalia that must be examined to determine virginity:

l. Condition of the Vulva

Normally the labia majora and minora are in close contact with one another covering almost completely the external genetalia. After defloration, the labia may gape exposing the introitus vulvae.

The finding may not be relied upon because some females may have inherently gaping labia, especially, asthenic women although there is no history of previous sexual act, While others may "preserve the coaptated labia even if there had been previous sexual acts.

2. Fourchette

The normal V-shape of the fourchette is lost on account of the previous stretching during insertion of the male organ. Withdrawal of the stretching force will cause retraction of its walls with rounding of the lower portion of the base;

Retraction of the fourchette is not a good sign of defloration inasmuch as it can be due to some causes. Ballet dancing, separation of the thighs, tree climbing, cycling, horse riding, insertion of foreign body, etc. may cause retraction of the fourchette without previous sexual act.

The fourchette, together with the perineum and lower portion of the posterior vaginal wall, may be lacerated by sexual act or some other causes.

3. Vaginal Canal

After repeated sexual acts, there is diminution of the sharpness or obliterations of the vaginal rugosities. There will be laxity of its wall so that insertion of a medium size tube during the medical examination can be done with slight resistance.

The changes in the vaginal rugosities or the laxity of its wall cannot be relied upon as a proof of defloration because instrument during medical examination, masturbation or insertion of foreign bodies or other similar or related acts will cause the development of such condition.

The vaginal wall, together with the vulva, may suffer injury during defloration of some other cause.

Causes of Vulvo-Vaginal Injuries

The following are the predisposing causes of vulvo-vaginal injuries during sexual act.

1. Virginity - sex organ does not have previous experience to stretching or coital
2. Pre-puberty – the genital organ is not yet fully developed to subject it to full physiological function.
3. Genital disproportion the male organ is unusually big or female organ infantile in size in spite of adult age.
4. Unprepared or un aroused female - the vaginal -secretion is absent, causing more friction.
5. Position during the sexual act - doral decubitus position with the thighs hypeflexed predisposes to deep penetration by the male organ and is contributory to vaginal vault laceration. The vaginal position may not be in harmony with the movement of the penis the sexual attack or intercourse.

6. Brutality of the male partner during the sexual act, recent vaginal surgery- the canal may become narrow and fibrous scar may replace the muscular vaginal wall at the site of surgery, and excessive active involvement of the female partner.
7. Multiple sexual act among sex deviates or multiple consort continuous stretching and friction may weaken its wall, renewed sexual activity after prolonged abstinence, post-menopause, and uterine retroversion.

4. Hymen

The hymen is lacerated during the initial sexual act. However, it is not always the case. Some hymen is thick, elastic and ûeshy such that they can resist certain degree of distention without causing laceration. Some women may inherently have lacerated hyrnen probably on account of previous trauma during the early age. The fact that the hymen is intact does not prove absence of previous sexual intercourse and the presence of laceration does not provide defloration.

The other causes of hymenal laceration are as follows: passage of clotted blood; ulceration due to disease, like diphtheria, jumping or running; falling on hard and sharp object, medical instrumentation, self-scratching due to irritation, masturbation, insertion of foreign bodies, previous operation; and local medication.

Inclusion in the Examination of the Hymen

Hereunder are some of the important considerations in the inclusion of hymen during the conduct of medico-legal examination, as follows:

1. General Condition of the Hymen

This includes the width, thickness, elasticity, vascularity, and laxity. It may include pathological condition, like inflammatory changes, signs of previous trauma, developmental of abnormality, and presence of foreign elements.

2. Original Shape of the Orifice

In case of laceration is present, try to reconstruct the hymen by means of probe and determine the original shape of the opening. It may linear, circular, stellate, cresentic, septate, cribform, imperforate and fimbriated.

3. Presence of Laceration

If there is presence of laceration, the following must be noted:

a. Degree of Laceration

This refers to the extent of damage to the hymen which may be:

1. Incomplete Laceration rupture or laceration of the hymen is considered incomplete when it does not involve the whole width or height of the hymen. Incomplete laceration may be:
2. Superticial laceration - the laceration does not go beyond one- half of the whole width of the hymen.
3. Deep -the laceration involves more than one-half of the width of the hymen but not reaching the base.

b. Complete Laceration

The hymenal laceration involves the whole Width but not beyond the base of the hymen.

c. Compound of Complicated Laceration

The laceration involves the hymen and also the surrounding tissues. It may involve the perineum, vaginal canal, utherta or rectum.

d. Location of Laceration

For the purpose of locating the site of the laceration, the hymenal orifice is related to the face of watch while the subject is in lithonomy position. With the examiner facing the female genitalia, the location of the laceration will be described corresponding to the time in the face of watch.

By this, a laceration at the region of fourchette may be described as a laceration at 6:00 o'clock position in the face of a watch, while on the horizontal sides may be termed 9:00 o'clock – left side and 3:00 o'clock light side.

e. Duration of the Laceration

The determination as to how long the laceration took place can be approximated by the changes observed in the lacerated tissue.

1. Flesh bleeding laceration - the laceration is of recent origin.
2. Fresh healing laceration - usually after twenty-four hours.
3. Healed laceration with congested edges and with sharp coaptible border depending upon the degree of laceration and the presence or the absence of complications, the said laceration could occur four to ten days. Sometimes, said finding is termed recently healed laceration.
4. Healed laceration with sharp coaptible borders without congestion - sometimes have passed by after the laceration-has healed. Ordinarily it can be inferred that hymenal laceration took place approximately more than ten days or two to three weeks.
5. Healed Laceration with Rounded Non-Coaptible Borders and Retraction of Edges - laceration took place long before the date of the examination is probably more than month's time.

f. Complications of Laceration

A vast majority of laceration of the hymen healed uneventfully, although in rare instances complications set in. The following are the possible complications:

1. Secondary infection- there may be activation of the bacterial flora in the vaginal canal or a superimposed infection may set in, especially among women with poor hygienic habit. Gonorrheal infection is not uncommon when the offender is suffering from the disease at the time of sexual attack;
2. Hemorrhage - this is a rare complication but this may be present m severe compound laceration of the hymen. Surgical intervention may be necessary to control the bleeding, Blood analysis to determine the presence of blood disease may be indicated when there is disproportion between the injury and the amount of hemorrhage. Blood transfusion may be required when the condition of the patient demands replacement of the blood loss.
3. Fistulae Formation - recto-vaginal or vesico-vaginal fistula may develop in case of compound laceration, This may require the services of a competent gynecologist to subject the patient to surgery.

4. Stricture - hymenal laceration alone will not produce stricture but in case of involvement of the vaginal wall it may consequently result in narrowing of the canal on account of the scar formation.
5. Sterility - trauma and infection may further involve the. Upper part of the female generative organ and may loss of procreation power.

Death Related to Sexual-Acts

Hereunder are some causes of death related to sexual acts:

l. Death of the Male Partner

a. Death from natural cause

During the sexual intercourse, the male as an active subject develops increase in blood pressure, tachycardia and hyper-ventilation due to emotional response and muscular exertion, If he is suffering from cardio-vascular disease or insufficiency of cardiac reserve, the increase demand on the cardio- vascular system may not be met, hence may die, this is also true in masturbation.

b. Death Due to the defensive act of the victim

In cases of rape, the victim may be able to take hold of a sharp instrument and inflict injuries to the offender which may cause his death.

2. Death of the Female Partner

Women almost never suffer death from natural causes during the normal sexual act. The reason maybe they are less susceptible to cardio-vascular disease and that they play a passive role ill sexual intercourse.

Women can control their tendencies to over-excitement and they exert less physical effort in a sexual act than men do. Death of the female partner is usually accidental and not on account of a natural disease.

a. The sexual intercourse might be done in a relatively confined space like the back seat of the car. Accidental strangulation or suffocation of the female partner may be due to the undue pressure applied on the chest, neck or face. The struggle of the female partner may remain unnoticed on account of the height of sexual excitement, and this may cause her death.

b. In case of oral sex wherein the male penis is placed in the mouth of the female partner, the size and length of the penis may cause partial or total block of the air passage, causing asphyxia. Ejaculation of seminal fluid may occlude the lumen of the respiratory tract as in drowning.

c. In case of cunnilingus, the male partner may blow air in the vulva and may cause air embolism, especially when the woman is pregnant. The air may enter the blood circulation and causes immediate death.

d. Sadists who may not be sexually satisfied by sexual intercourse. But by inflicting physical injuries to the partner may cause death of the female partner.

e. Death of the female partner may be deliberately done by the male to conceal the crime of rape he has committed. The male partner inflict physical injuries, or may cause asphyxiation by strangulation or by other means.

f. The female partner may die of shock as a result of extreme physical and mental trauma in case of rape, hemorrhage and infection due to sexually transmitted disease.

3. Death of Both Partners

Almost simultaneous death of both partners during sexual intercourse maybe due to the performance of the sexual act in an enclosed place with carbon monoxide or other asphyxiate gas. Examination of their respective blood will reveal the presence of gas incompatible with life; and homicide-suicide pact.

Medical Evidences in the Crime of Rape

Hereunder are the most common medical evidences in the crime of rape:

1. Evidence from the Victim

Before actual examination is made on the subject, it is necessary to have a written consent may be subject herself of from her guardian, if the victim is not of age. If the woman is conûned in a correctional institution the consent may be given by the head of the institution.

A short history of the alleged rape must be taken and it is advisable to reduce it writing. The history must include all the circumstances leading to the abuse, the age of the victim at the time of the alleged commission of the offense and also the menstrual history.

It may be used as guide to the examining physician to the different points that must be emphasized in the course of the examination. Aside from the history, the following points must be also recorded by the physician:

a. Date, time and place of alleged rape

This is necessary in. order to determine how long a time has elapsed after alleged commission of the offense before the victim filed the necessary complaint or subjected herself to the medical-legal examination.

If several days have gone by before the filing of the complaint, let her explain the cause of the delay. The place where the alleged offense was committed is necessary to determine which court can acquire jurisdiction over the case.

b. Date, time and place of the examination

The date of the physical examination is material to the determination of the possible findings of the physician on the victim. A long interval of time between the date of commission and the examination will remove the possibility of finding the effects of a recent sexual attack or intercourse.

c. Condition of the clothing

If force is applied in the commission of the offense, there will be tearing, staining with blood and semen, and soiling of the clothing. The clothing must be preserved after they have been thoroughly dried for further laboratory examination.

d. Gait, facial expression, body and attitude

The physician must observe the gait, the facial expression and the bodily and mental attitude of the subject. If the victim suffered from genital injuries she may walk with legs apart and slowly, with the face manifesting signs that she is suffering from pain.

e. Physical and mental development of victim

The height strength and degree of muscular development of the woman must be noted to determine whether she has the capacity to resists any unlawful aggression.

i. If the victim is a child, examination of the physical condition is not necessary because it is apparent to the age. In most cases, children are bribed or lured by attractive articles such. As candies by the offender.

The examiner must observe the mental state of the victim. She may be in the state of mental shock, under influence of depressant drugs, alcohol or sex stimulants; The offender might have taken advantage of her insanity or mental deficiency. The victim may appear exhausted, despondent or account of the public humiliation she will suffer, or maybe hostile to the investigator. Care and more psychological approach are necessary in order to get the full cooperation and consent.

f. Examination of body for signs of violence

If actual force was applied in the commission of the crime, there must be signs of physical violence on the body of the victim. Her whole body must be subjected to inspection. Physical injuries must be described and the exact location must be determined. Areas of tenderness or swelling must not be over looked and if necessary X-Ray pictures must be taken to determine bone lesions.

g. Examination of the genitalia and breast

The breast must be examined for the presence of finger mark or application of pressure. They might have been roughly handled or the nipples bitten. The vulva may show swelling, tenderness, contusion, abrasion, laceration or may be smeared with blood semen and other foreign bodies.

The hymen may show fresh laceration, swelling or bruising, There may be healed laceration or signs of physical virginity. In the pubic hair, the following medical evidence may be gathered, i.e., pubic hair of the offender; semen and spermatozoa, blood stains and body louse.

Abrasion which is normally found in the posterior commeasure is usually brought about by friction or a violent attempt of insert. The vaginal canal may show obliteration of the rugosities or even purulent discharge.

2. Examination of the Alleged Offenders

a. Physical development, mental and strength

The relative physical development and strength of the victim and the offender must be compared to determine whether the offender can overpower the resistance offered by the victim;

b. Evidence of physical injuries

The whole body must be examined. The victim, in the course of struggle, may inflict bodily harm to the offender. Fingernail marks on the neck, arms and chest may be found. The fermium of the penis may be abraded or lacerated on account of the violent insertion on a relatively small vulgar or vaginal opening.

c. Condition of the sex organ

Aside from the examination of the fermium, washing from the surface of the penis may reveal blood, seminal stain, vaginal epithelium and orderlies bacillus. The urethral meat us may be moist on account of the recent discharge.

d. Evidence from the pubic hair

The pubic hair may be matted together due to blood stains or from seminal fluid discharge. Examine carefully for the presence of body locus.

e. Potency of the offender

The offender my put up a defense that he -is impotent arid that it could have been hardly possible that he had committed the crime. It may be necessary to subject the offender to strong sex stimulation sufficiently under normal condition to produce erection.

f. Evidence from genital infection

If the offender is suffering from venereal disease which is transmitted to the victim during the criminal act, the crime committed is rape with physical injuries because infection in raw is physical injuries.

3. Evidence from the Companion of the Victim

a. A history of the incident must be taken front the companion of the victim.

   Try to see whether there are consistent with narration of facts by the victim.

b. If the companion helped the victim when force was applied by the offender, the companion must be subjected to a physical and medical examination for physical injuries.

c. Examination of the clothing may be necessary for signs of struggle.

d. Investigation must be made to determine whether the companion might have participated as an accomplice to the crime.

e. The mental condition, physical power, age, and emotional state must be taken into consideration to determine the capacity to resist unlawful aggression from the offender.

f. Examination must be made as to the presence of alcohol or other depressant which may diminish the companion's capacity to defend the victim from the offender.

9

Medico Legal Aspects of Abortion

The Medical Termination of Pregnancy (MTP) Act of India 1971 states the conditions under which a pregnancy can be ended or aborted, the persons who are qualified to conduct the abortion and the place of implementation.

Some of these qualifications are as follows:

a. Women whose physical and/or mental health were endangered by the pregnancy.

b. Women facing the birth of a potentially handicapped or malformed child.

c. Rape.

d. Pregnancies in unmarried girls under the age of eighteen with the consent of a guardian.

e. Pregnancies in "lunatics" with the consent of a guardian.

f. Pregnancies that are a result of failure in sterilization.

Abortion in India is legal only up to twenty weeks of pregnancy under specific conditions and situations, which are broadly defined as:

1. the continuance of the pregnancy would involve a risk to the life of the pregnant woman or of grave injury of physical or mental health, or

2. there is a substantial risk that if the child were born, it would suffer from such physical or mental abnormalities as to be seriously handicapped.

Recently, the Supreme Court permitted a rape survivor to terminate her pregnancy at 24 weeks, which is beyond the permissible 20 weeks limit prescribed under the Medical Termination of Pregnancy Act, 1971.

Definition of Abortion

Abortion is defined as the termination of pregnancy by the removal or expulsion from the uterus of a fetus or embryo prior to viability. An abortion can occur spontaneously or accidentally, in which case it is usually called miscarriage or unintentional abortion, or it can be purposely induced. The term abortion most commonly refers to the induced. abortion of a human pregnancy.

Different Types of Abortion

Enumerated and briefly discusses hereunder are the different types of abortions, as follows:

1. Induced

Most abortions result from unintended pregnancies A pregnancy be intentionally aborted in several ways. The manner selected often depends upon the gestational age of the embryo or fetus, which increases in size as the pregnancy progresses. Specific procedures may also be selected due to legality, regional, availability, and doctor or patient preferences.

2. Spontaneous

Spontaneous abortion, also known as miscarriage, is the unintentional expulsion of an embryo or fetus before the 24th Week of gestation. A pregnancy that ends before 37 weeks of gestation resulting in a live born infant is known as a 'premature birth' or a 'preterm birth'. When a fetus dies in uterus after viability, or during delivery, it is usually termed 'stillborn abortion'.

Categories of Induced Abortion

Briefly discussed hereunder are the numerous categories of induced abortion, as follows:

1. Medical

Medical abortions are those induced by abortifacient pharmaceuticals.

2. Surgical

Gestation, suction aspiration or vacuum aspiration is the most common surgical methods of induced abortion. Manual vacuum aspiration consists of removing the fetus by suction using a manual syringe, while electric vacuum aspiration uses an electric pump. These techniques differ in the in the mechanism used to apply suction, in how early in pregnancy they can be used, and in whether cervical dilation is necessary.

3. Other Methods

Historically, a number of herbs reputed to possess abortifacient properties were used. The use of herbs in such a planner can cause serious even lethal side effects, such as multiple organ failure, and is not recommended by physicians. Abortion is sometimes attempted by causing trauma to the abdomen, misoprostol, and insertion of non surgical implements such as knitting needles and clothes hangers into the uterus.

Varied Types of Clinical Abortion

Hereunder are the varied types of clinical abortion, as follows:

1. Missed abortion - an ovum destroyed by haemorrhage into the choriospace, usually before the fourth month of pregnancy. The hemorrhage takes place from maternal sinuses into the decidus.
2. Threatened abortion - haemorrhage without dilatation of the internal os. Haemorrhage in early stage of pregnancy may be due to causes other than threatened abortion, e.g., ectopic pregnancy, and cervical polyp.
3. Inevitable abortion - haemorrhage with dilatation of the internal os and presence of rhythmical pain. It may end by the spontaneous expulsion of the product of conception or may requires intervention.

4. Incomplete abortion - not all the product of misconception has been expelled from the uterus, fragments or portions of which is retained. This will prevent contraction of uterus and consequently uncontrolled- bleeding will develop.
5. Complete abortion - the whole product of conception is expelled, and the fetus died after its expulsion. All the parties involved in the commission of the criminal act can be held criminally liable.

Medical Evidences of Abortion

Hereunder are important considerations in the collection of medical evidences relatively with the crime of abortion as follows:

1. Medical Evidence in the Living

a. Presence of external signs of violence in the form of contusions, abrasions, hematoma, open wounds or whatever form on the body surface if induced by general violence. If evidence is applied locally in the generative tract, injuries or whatever form on description may be seen therein.

b. Examination of the generative tract;

1. appearance of the external genitalia and vagina may show laceration, contusion, abrasions, and other marks of instrumentation.
2. examine the external genitalia and vagina for softness, tear, and discharge.
3. note the size of the uterus, its consistency, and laceration.

c. Examination of the instrument

uses for the presence of blood, placental tissue or fetal parts, and note the history of health beforehand after abortion and history of having ingested or injected with abortive drugs.

d. Signs of previous pregnancy are as follows:

1. conditions of the breasts.
2. laxity of the abdominal wall.
3. paleness of integument, general body weakness, presence of characteristic lochial discharge and odor.

4. palpability of the uterus and laceration of the cervix and perineum.

e. Laboratory test for pregnancy

test and testimony of the physician who completed the abortion or of other persons who witnesses the criminal act.

f. Examination of the expelled product of conception as follows:

1. blood examination maternity and paternity.
2. marks of instrumentation.
3. signs of physical violence.
4. proof of viability or non-viability of the fetus.
5. presence of abortive and other toxic materials in the fetal blood.
6. presence or absence of malformation.
7. completeness of the placenta.
8. other identifying marks.

Medical Evidence in the Dead

Aside from the evidences of abortion in the living which may be found in the dead, the following may be observed at autopsy:

a. Evidence of instrumentation. This will include the presence of punctured wounds in the placenta, presence or remnants of the placenta inside the uterine cavity, and presence of perforations in the uterus.

b. Examination of stomach and its contents. Abortifacient drugs of any kinds and other irritants may be found inside the stomach upon chemical examination.

c. Examination of the uterine contents. Remnant of the product of conception must be examined for the following:

1. infection, 2. stage of pregnancy, and 3. other complication of abortion.

d. Examination of the kidneys and other organs for irritants. Like the stomach and its contents, other organs like the kidneys, liver, spleen must be subjected to qualitative chemical examination for the presence of irritant poisons.

e. Examination of some untoward effects of abortions, such as follows:

1. infection, toxemia, or bacteremia, 2. embolism, 3. fistulae formation, and 4. pelvic adhesion.

f. Biological test such as follows: paternity test and test for pregnancy.

Post-Mortem Abortion

This is the expulsion of the products of conception after death of the pregnant woman brought about by the post-mortem contraction of the uterine muscles. It is possible during the early stage of pregnancy when the fetus, is small. During the later stage, the contraction of the uterus may cause its rupture and expel as contents of pregnancy into the abdominal cavity.

10
Forensic Pathology

Medico legal investigation of death is the most crucial and significant of the medical examiner. The medical is primarily concerned determining the cause and manner of death, identifying the deceased, determining the approximate time of death and injury, collecting evidence, and documenting these events through an official autopsy report. The basis of the medico-legal investigation is forensic pathology.

What is Pathology?

Pathology is derived from the Greek words pathos, meaning suffering and logos meaning discourse" or study. It is the science or study of disease. A pathologist studies the cause or nature of the diseases and identifies the changes diseases create in the human body.

Definition of Forensic Pathology

Forensic pathology is a branch of pathology which is concerned with determining the cause of death by examination of a corpse. The autopsy is performed by the pathologist at the request of medical examiner usually during the conduct of scientific investigation, Whether it is either criminal cases or civil disputes.

Branches of Forensic Pathology

The two main branches of forensic pathology are as follows:

1. *Anatomic Pathology*

This branch of pathology deals with the evaluation of tissues that is obtained from living or dead people with the help of the microscope. The main subcategories of anatomic pathology are autopsy, surgical and cytopathology. The surgical pathologist examines tissues and organs with the aim of making a diagnosis for any disease.

2. Clinical Pathology

This branch of pathology involves the evaluation of body fluids with the help of the laboratory. The main sub categories of clinical pathology are hematology, microbiology, chemistry hematology and immunology. Among the forensic pathologists the branches of chemistry and toxicology are the most popular.

Scope of Forensic Pathology

Forensic pathology is an application of medical jurisprudence. The scope of forensic pathology is broad and encompassing, as follows:

1. The forensic pathologist is a medical doctor who has completed training in anatomical pathology and who has subsequently sub specialized in forensic pathology, who examines and documents wounds and injuries, both at autopsy and occasionally in a clinical setting.
2. Performs postmortem examinations to determine the cause of death. The autopsy report contains an opinion about, i.e., the pathologic process, injury, or disease that directly results in or initiates a series of events which lead to a person's death, and the circumstances surrounding the cause of death.
3. Collects and examines tissue specimens under the microscope in order to identify the presence or absence of natural disease and other microscopic findings, and collects and interprets toxicological analyses on body tissues and fluids to determine the chemical cause of accidental overdoses or deliberate poisonings.
4. The autopsy also provides an opportunity for other issues raised by the death to be addressed, such as the collection of trace evidence or determining the identity of the deceased.
5. Forensic pathologists also work closely with the medico-legal authority for the area concerned with the investigation of

sudden and unexpected deaths; and serves as an expert witness in courts of law testifying in civil or criminal law cases.

Forensic physicians, sometimes referred to as forensic medical examiners or police surgeons are medical doctors trained the examination of, and provision of medical treatment to, living victims of assault and those individuals who find themselves in police custody.

Roles of Forensic Pathologist

The role of a forensic pathologist was to determine the cause, mechanism manner of death, takes a deep knowledge of human anatomy, physiology and pathology. Pathologists are doctors of medicine that study the diseases affecting the human body, with specialized entities responsible for conducting autopsies.

The forensic pathologist deals with the study of medicine as it applies to criminal law, in addition, the forensic pathologist is more likely to do with physical injuries. More than fifty percent of the time participated in causing the death by the outbreak of the diseases. The forensic pathologist is qualified to perform medico-legal autopsies, and proof of performance must testify in open court as his professional opinion.

The forensic pathologist is at the top of the pyramid system of forensic investigations. However the work of the profession, not all are clean and tidy as a desk job all day, as pushing pencils. This work requires bodily fluids of a deceased person exposed to odors, and disease. It can also be rewarding, fascinating, and intellectually stimulating.

The job description also includes the support of the support of the right law enforcement agencies with search and recovery procedures of the body and providing advice in criminal court. He has a vast knowledge human anatomy, physiology, pathology, anthropology, dental, microscopy X-1 rules and test evidence, crime scene assessment and rules on evidence.

Concern of Forensic Pathology

Forensic pathology is concerned with analyzing medical evidence in crimes. This is done by the examination of the body at autopsy of tissues removed during surgery, and by analysis of fluids from the body, such as blood or urine, in the clinical pathology laboratory. The forensic pathologists involvement and investigation includes visiting the scene of death. Gathering information about what happened at the time and place of the subject's death, what he or she was doing, and the health of health is of vital importance.

The forensic examination of the body includes examining the clothing on the body, the body itself, and the internal examination of the organs in the body, which is the autopsy. The autopsy may include microscopic and x-ray examinations of the tissues of the body. The forensic pathologist may call in many others in his search for answers. Evidence such as fingernail clippings and scrapings in an assault case, swabs. For examination for sperm and seminal fluid, hair samples, and ûbers on the deceased's clothing and body are sent to a crime laboratory for a criminalist to study.

Autopsy ûndings must be correlated with information about the events surrounding the death and the place where death occurred. Examination of the body might indicate that death did. not occur where or in the position the body was found; the body may have been moved after the death. The forensic pathologist and the autopsy are vital parts of p1opei medico-legal death investigation. The forensic scientists must work without bias, This work may lead to the conviction of an assailant, or it may protect an innocent person. The forensic pathologist must give dispositions and must testify court about the autopsy findings and toxicological results in law suits.

Forensic Pathology Process

The purpose of an autopsy is to observe and make a permanent legal record as soon as possible of the gross and minute anatomical peculiarities of a recently discovered dead body. Autopsies are typically done at a hospital. Anatomic examination may be sufficient to establish cause of death if the forensic pathologist has access to other information.

Forensic pathologists also sometimes engage in psychological autopsies although these are not all that readily accepted by the legal system. Clinical or microscopic, examination of organ parts is often necessary to further bolster the forensic pathologists conclusions, although such examination would be impossible in an examination case since embalming -usually thwarts the microscopic laboratory and criminalistic testing.

Forensic pathologists almost always order x-ray examination whenever firearm is involved. X-rays are also sometimes useful in stab wound and child abuse cases. The examination of organ parts from the body is useful in toxicology cases as well as anytime alcohol or drugs are suspected. The inspection of stomach contents is part of every postmortem exam since it may provide information as to cause of death as well as time of death. Clinical examination also tends to confirm hunches about age, race, sex height weight and general condition in cases of unidentified remains.

Autopsies are highly specialized procedures performed for various purposes and can range from external examination to internal examination In the case of internal examination, the body is reconstituted by sewing it back together. About 25% of the time, autopsy will reveal a different cause of death than the one everyone believes is the cause of death of the victim.

Besides cause of death, attempts will be made to estimate time of death and what, if anything preceded the death. Once a body is received it is photograph applied, has its clothes removed, and is then subjected to ultraviolent light. Samples of hair and nails are taken, and the body is then cleaned, weighed, and measured before any incisions are made for internal examination.

Significance of Forensic Pathology

Leading forensic pathologists from around the world synthesize the practical advances in a variety of important sub-specialties of forensic pathology and demonstrate how the latest medical and scientific progress is being applied to solve current problems of high interest to forensic pathologists today. Forensic pathology offers cutting-edge insights into death from environmental conditions, homicide by sharp force, death from natural causes, and pathology of human endotheliuni in septic organ failure.

Special aspects of crime scene interpretation and behavioral analysis, neo- genesis of ethanol and fuel oils in putrefying blood, agrochemical poisoning, imaging techniques in forensic pathology and fixation techniques for organs and parenchymal structures. The forensic pathologists involvement and investigation includes visiting the scene of death. Gathering information about what happened at the time and place of the subjects death, what he or she was doing, and the health of the subject is of vital importance.

The forensic examination of the body includes examining the clothing on the body, the body itself, and the internal examination of the organs in the body, which is the autopsy. The autopsy may include microscopic and x-ray examinations of the tissues of the body. The forensic pathologist may call in many others in his search for answers, and must "determine which injuries were received when the victim was alive, which changes occurred after death, and which injuries were received after death.

11
Forensic Entomology

The study of insect activity on cadavers yields important clues about the date and the location of death. Determining the date and location are very important to homicide investigations; knowing when and where a person dies can mean the difference between solving a crime and watching a case grow cold. Proving where and when a victim died can help lead investigators in convicting or releasing a suspect.

Definition of Forensic Entomology

It is the application and study of insect and other arthropod biology to criminal matters. Forensic entomology is primarily associated with death investigations; however, it may also be used to detect drugs and poisons, determine the location of an incident, and find the presence and time of the infliction of wounds.

Medico-Legal Forensic Entomology Definition

Medico-legal forensic entomology covers evidence gathered through arthropod studies at the scenes of murder, suicide, rape, physical abuse and contraband trafficking. In murder investigations it deals with which insect eggs appear, their location on the body and in what order they appear.

This can be helpful in determining a post mortem interval (PMI) and location of a death in question. Since many insects exhibit a degree of endemism occurring only in certain places, or have a well-defined phenology active only at a certain season, or time of day, their presence in association with other evidence can demonstrate potential links to times and locations where other events may have occurred.

Another area covered by medico-legal forensic entomology is the relatively new field of entomo-toxicological. This particular branch involves the utilization of entomological specimens found at a scene in order to test for different drugs that in ay have possibly played a role in the death of the victim.

Using Insects to Determine Post-Mortem Interval

By the 1800's, scientists knew that certain insects would inhabit decomposing bodies. Interest now turned to the matter of succession. Physicians and legal investigators began questioning which insects would appear first on a cadaver, and what their life cycles could reveal about a crime.

In 1855, French doctor Bergeret d'Arbois was the first to use insect succession to determine the postmortem interval of human remains. A couple remodeling their Paris home uncovered the in mummified remains of a child behind the mantelpiece. Suspicion immediately fell on the couple, though they had only recently moved in to the house.

Bergeret, who autopsied the victim, noted evidence of insect populations on the corpse. Using methods similar to those employed by forensic entomologists today, he concluded that the body had been placed behind the wall years earlier, in 1849. Bergeret used what was known about insect life cycles and successive colonization of a corpse to arrive at this date.

His report convinced police to charge the previous tenants of the home, who were subsequently convicted of the murder. French veterinarian Jean Pierre Megnin spent years studying and documenting the predictability of insect colonization in cadavers. In 1894, he published La: Fcizme des Cadavres, the culmination of his medico-legal experience.

In it, he outlined eight waves of insect succession that could be applied during investigations of suspicious deaths. Megnin also noted that buried corpses were not susceptible to this same series of colonization. Just two stages of colonization invaded these cadavers.

Information from the Death Scene

Forensic entomologists are commonly called upon to determine the postmortem interval or time since death in homicide investigations. More speciûcally, the forensic entomologist estimates a portion of the postmortem interval based on the age of the insect present. This entomological based estimation is most commonly called the time since colonization.

Based on the factors in a particular investigation, this may, or may not, closely approximate the entire postmortem interval. In either case, it is the duty of the Forensic Pathologist or Medical Examiner to estimate the postmortem interval and the Forensic Entomologist may assist them in providing information on the time since colonization which can ultimately be used to substantiate a portion of the postmortem interval.

The forensic entomologist can use a number of different techniques including species succession, larval weight, larval length, and a more technical method known as the accumulated degree hour technique which can be very precise if the necessary data is available. A qualified forensic entomologist can also make inferences as to possible postmortem improvement of a corpse. Some flies prefer specific habitats such as a distinct preference for laying their eggs in outdoor or indoor environment.

Flies can also exhibit preferences for carcasses in shade or sunlit conditions of the outdoor environment. Therefore, a corpse that is recovered indoors. with the eggs larvae of flies that typically inhabit sunny outdoor locations would indicate that someone returned to the scene of the crime to move and attempt to conceal the body. Similarly, freezing or wrapping of the body may be indicated by an altered species succession of insects on the body.

Anything that may have prevented the insects from laying eggs in their normal time frame will alter both the sequence of species and their typical colonization time. This alteration of the normal insect succession and fauna should be noticeable to the forensic entomologists if they are familiar with what would normally be recovered from a body in a particular environmental habitat or geographical location.

The complete absence of insects would suggest clues as to the sequence of postmortem events as the body was probably either frozen and sealed in a tightly closed container buried very deeply. Entomological evidence can also help determine the circumstances of abuse and rape. Victims that are incapacitated often have associated fecal and urine soaked clothes or bed dressings. Such material will attract certain species offices that otherwise would not be recovered.

Their presence can yield many clues to both ante-mortem and postmortem circumstances of the crime. Currently, it is now possible to use DNA technology not only to help determine insect species, but to recover and identify the blood meals taken by blood feeding insects. The DNA of human blood can be recovered from the digestive tract of an insect that has fed on an individual.

The presence of their DNA within the insect can place suspects at a known location within a deûnable period of time and recovery of the victims blood can also create a link between perpetrator and suspect. The insects recovered from decomposing human remains can be a valuable tool for toxicological analysis. The voracious appetite of the insects on corpses can quickly skeletonize the remains. In a short period of time the fluids and soft tissues needed for toxicological analysis disappear. However, it is possible to recover the insect larvae and run standard toxicological analyses on them as you would human tissue. Toxicological analysis can be successful on insect larvae because their tissues assimilate drugs and toxins that accumulated in human tissue prior to death.

How Insects Reveal the Time of Death

When a suspicious death occurs, a forensic entomologist may be called to assist in processing the crime scene. Insects found on or near the body may reveal important clues about the crime, including the victim's time or death. Insects colonize cadavers in a predictable sequence, also known as insect succession. The first to arrive are the necrophagous species, drawn by the strong scent of decomposition.

Blow flies can invade-a corpse within minutes of death and flesh flies follow close behind. Soon, after come the dermestid beetles, the same beetles used by taxidermists to clean skulls of their flesh. More flies gather, including house flies Predatory at parasitic insects arrive to feed on the maggots and beetle larvae. Eventually, as the corpse dries, hide beetles and clothes moths find the remains.

Forensic-entomologists collect samples of crime scene insects, making sure to take representatives of every species at their latest Stage of development. Because arthropod development is linked directly to temperature she also gathers daily temperature data from the nearest available weather station. In the lab, the scientist identities each insect to species, and determines their exact developmental stage. Since identification of maggots can be difficult, the Entomologist usually raises some of the maggots to adulthood to confirm their species.

Blow flies and flesh are the most useful crime scene insects for determining the post-mortem interval, or time of death. Through laboratory studies, scientists have established the developmental rates of necrophagous species, based on constant temperatures in a laboratory environmental. These databases relate a species life stage to its age when developing at a constant temperature, and provide the entomologist with a measurement called accumulated degree days, or ADD. ADD represents physiological time. Using the known ADD, forensic entomologist can then calculate the likely age of a specimen from the corpse, adjusting for the temperature and other environmental conditions present at the crime scene.

Working backwards through physiological time, the forensic entomologist can provide investigators with a specific time period the body was first colonized by necrophagous insects. Since, these insects almost always find the corpse within minutes or hours of the person's death, this calculation reveals the postmortem interval with good accuracy.

Use of Insects to Tell If a Body Was Moved

In some suspicious death investigations, arthropod evidence may prove that the body was moved at some point after death. Crime, scene insects can tell whether the body decomposed at the location where it was found, and even reveal gaps in the crime time line, as follows:

1. Crime scene insects inconsistent with the body's location

The entomologist first identifies all the collected arthropod evidence, cataloging the species present on or near the body. Not every insect belongs in every habitat. Some live in quite specific niches on limited vegetation types, at certain elevations, or in particular climates. What if the body yields an insect that is not known to live in the area where it was found? Wouldn't that suggest the body had been moved? In one such case, an investigator collected evidence from a woman's body found in a sugar called field. The investigator noted that some if the maggots present were a species of fly found in urban areas, not in agricultural fields. Then the investigator hypothesized that the body had remained in an urban location long enough for the flies to find it, and that it was later moved to the field. Sure enough, when the murder was solved, his theory proved correct.

2. Crime scene insects inconsistent with the crime timeline

Sometimes insect evidence reveals a gap in the time line, and leads investigators to the conclusion that the body was moved. The primary focus of forensic entomology is the establishment of the postmortem interval, using insect life cycles. A good forensic entomologist will give detectives an estimate, to the day or even the hour, of when the body was first colonized by insects. Investigators compare this estimate with Witness accounts of when the victim was last seen alive. Where was the victim between when he was last seen and when insects first invaded his corpse.

Here is a good; example of a case where insect evidence established such a time gap. A body found on August 8th yielded only first instant maggots, some still emerging from their eggs. Based on the criminal investigator is knowledge of this insects since life cycle in the environmental conditions present at the crime scene, concluded that the body had only been exposed to insects since the previous day, the 7th day.

According to available witnesses, the victim was last seen alive two days prior, on the 5 th day. It seemed that the body must live been somewhere else, protected from exposure to any insects, in the interim. In the end, the murderer was caught and revealed he had killed the victim on the 5 th day, but kept the body in the trunk of a car until finally deciding to dump it on the 7th day.

3. Crime scene insects in the soil

A dead body lying on the ground will release all its fluids into the soil below. As a result of this seepage, the soil chemistry changes substantially. Native soil organisms leave the area as the pH rises and the whole new community of particular types of anthropoids inhabits this gruesome niche. A forensic entomologist will sample the soil below and near where the body was lying.

The organisms found in the soil samples can determine whether the body decomposed at the location where it was found, or prior to being dumped there. What crime scene insects reveal about the victim's wounds by examining crime scene insects near or in wounds on a corpse, a forensic entomologist can usually distinguish which wounds occurred before or after the victim's death.

4. Insects on wounds inflicted prior to the victims death

When the heart is still beating, scratches, stab wounds, or bullet entries and exits will all bleed. Fresh, wet blood attracts necrophagous insects.

Insects will begin to feed and lay eggs in these open wounds, which provide them additional points of entry into the body.

5. Insects on wounds inflicted after the victims death

Postmortem wounds, on the other hand, tend not to bleed and often remain dry and clean. Insects are much less likely to enter. Body through wounds. delivered after the heart has stopped beating, causing the loss of tone of blood.

6. How a forensic entoinologist interprets insects on a wound

If a wound shows evidence of early and active infestation, the forensic entomologist may report this as an ante-mortem wound. A wound absent of maggots or other nechophagous insects is most likely a post-mortem wound.

Insect Types Useful in Forensic Entomology

There are many different types of insect studied in forensic entomology. The order in which insects feed on a corpse is known as faunal succession.

1. Flies or Order Diptera

These are often the first to arrive on the crime scene. They prefer a moist corpse for their offspring-maggots to feed on. The most significant types of fly include:

a. Blow Flies or Calliphoridae - this is often metallic in appearance, commonly known as bluebottles, greenbottles and blowflies. There are over 1500 species in the world and 38 British species. The adults range in length from 5 - 15 mm. Many in this family are attracted to rotting flesh, and can detect the smell of decay within minutes after death. Because most of the larvae feed on vertebrate carrion, species in this family have become very important in forensic entomology as the rates of developments of the larvae of different species can indicate the time of death. Blowfly larvae are also used in medicine in 'maggot therapy' where they are used to clean up wounds. The greenbottle Lucilia sericata is the most commonly used species. Anglers also use blowfly larvae as bait.

b. Flesh Flies or Sarcophagidae flesh flies, being viviparous, frequently give birth to live young on corpses of human and other animals, at any stage of decomposition from newly dead through to bloated or decaying through the latter is more common.

c. House Flies or Muscidae - it is the most common of all flies found in homes, indeed one of the most widely distributed insects; it is often considered a pest that can carry serious diseases. Each female fly can lay up to 500 eggs in several batches of about 751-to 150 eggs;

d. Cheese Flies or Piophilidae - this fly's larva infests cured meats, smoked fish, cheeses, and decaying animals and is sometimes called the cheese skipper for its leaping ability. Forensic entomology uses the presence of Piophila case larvae to help estimate the date of death for human remains.

e. Others - the other types of flies are as follows: coffin flies phoridae, lesser corpse flies sphaerocer.i.dae, lesser house flies fannidae, black scavenger flies - sepsidae, sun ûies - heleomyzidae, and black soldier fly stratiomiyidae, and the humpbacked flies-prohidae.

2. Beetles or Order Coleoptera

They are generally found on the corpse when it is more decomposed. In drier conditions, the beetles can be replaced by moth flies psychodidae; These are the types:

a. Rove Beetles or Staphylinidae - are elongate beetles with small elytra (Wing covers) and large jaws. Like other beetles inhabiting carrion, they have fast larval development with only three larval stages. They lay their eggs in the corpse, and the emerging larvae are also predator.

b. Hister Beetles or Histeridae - adult histerids are usually shiny beetles which have an introverted head. The carrion-feeding species only become active at night when they enter the maggot infested part of the corpse to capture and devour their maggot prey.

c. Carrion Beetles or Silphidae - adult Silphidae have an average size of about 12 mm. They are also referred to as burying beetles because they and bury small carcasses underground. Both parents tend to their young and exhibit communial breeding.

d. Scarab Beetles or Scarabaeidae scarab beetles may be any one of around 30,000 beetle species worldwide that are compact, heavy bodied and oval in shape. The flattened plates, which each antenna are fitted together to form a club.

3. Mites

Many mites or c1ass Acari feed on corpses with Macrochele mites common in the early stages of decomposition, while

Tyroglyphidae and Oribatidae mites such as Rostrozetes feed on dry skin in the later stages of decomposition.

4. Moths

Moths or Lepidoptera specifically clothes-moths are closely related to butterflies. Most species of moth are nocturnal, but I there are crepuscular and diurnal species. Moths feed mammalian hair daring their larval stages and may forage on any hair that remains on a body.

5. Wasps, Ants, and Bees

Wasps, ants, and bees or Hymenoptera are not necessarily necrophagous. While some feed on the body, some are also predatory, and eat the insects. feeding on the body. Bees and wasps have been seen feeding on the body during the early stages.

a. Wasps - Wasps exhibit a range of social difficulty, from private living to eusocial colonies. The non-breeding creatures care for the young or defend and supply for the group. Wasps are recommended for studies of evolutionary origin and maintenance of social behavior in animals;

b. Ants - among the most damaging of introduced species are ants. Many ants share some characteristic that ease their preamble, institution, and subsequent range expansion. One feature of their importance is the ability to establish numerically large, ecologically dominant colonies.

c. Bees - forensic entomologists have used bees in several cases where parents have used bees to sting their children as a form of discipline. Also, entomologists have been called upon to determine whether or not bees or wasps have been the cause of an accident.

Finding the Cause of Death Using Entomology

In a crime investigation, there is not only of great interest to find out when a victim died, but also of interest to find out how the victim died, as this can be used to find the killer. In some instances the insects themselves are the killers, in other instances the insects occurring on the carrion can shed a light on what happened when the victim died.

Wasps, and bees, for example, can inject venom through a sting. Some people are sensitive and allergic to these venoms, and can die if not treated in time. One other important aspect of wasps and bees are their effect on drivers. Many car accidents are probably caused by some; wasp, bee or bumble becoming through the window, causing hysteria, or a distraction from the road leading to a collision or other accidents. In some cases wasps and bees has been used as murder weapons, as if case where some parents had shut their infant in a room full of Wasps, in order to get rid of it.

Poison -can be traced in blood, urine, stomach contents, hair and nails. One other important source is maggots occurring on a corpse. After a while it will be impossible to sample stomach contents, urine and blood from the dead body, but it will still be possible to sample from maggots, empty puparia or larval skin cast. The following list of chemicals can be traced in maggots.

Many of these chemicals will also influence the life-cycle of the maggot. For example will high dosages of cocaine accelerate the development of some sarcophagus. Few insecticides are commonly used in suicide, and are usually taken orally. Presence of such insecticides in the mouth may lead to a delay in the colonization of the mouth. Presence of amitriptyline, an antidepressant, can prolong the developmental time with up to 77 hours, at least in one species of Sarcophagidae.

Knowledge of drug use in the victim is therefore important not only in finding the death cause, but also in estimating the time of death. The sites of blow fly infestation on the corpse maybe important ill determining the cause of death, or at least in reconstruction of events prior to death. For example; if there have been trauma, or mutilation of the body prior to death, this may lead to heavy infestation of other body parts than the usual sites when the victim is not mutilated.

Under a knife attack, it is usual to guard oneself with arms in front of thorax and head. This may lead to injury on the lower patt of the arm. After death, blow fly may oviposit in these wounds. The usual sites of oviposition on dead humans are natural openings Even here there is preference; blow flies will most often lay their eggs in the facial region, and more seldom in the genitoanal region. If there is a sexual assault prior to death, leading to bleeding in the genitoanal region, blowflies will be more likely to oviposit in these regions.

Therefore, if there is observed blowfly activity in the genitoanal region, one can start to suspect a sexual crime. This must of course be corroborated with other evidence as well. The interpretation of maggots in the anogenital region becomes very fuzzy after after (4-5) days, as eggs will be oviposited in this region during the course of decay in the natural course of decomposition.

Estimating Time of Death with Entomology

After the initial decay, and the body begins to smell, different types of insects are attracted to the dead body. The insects that usually arrives first is the Diptera, in particular the blow flies or Calliphoridae and the flesh flies or Sarcophagidae.

The females will lay their eggs on the body, especially around the natural orifices such as the nose, eyes and ears. If the body has wounds the eggs are also laid in such. Flesh flies do not lay eggs, but deposits larvae instead. After some short time, depending on species, the egg hatches into small larvae instead.

This larvae lives on the dead-tissue and grows fast. After a little time the 1arva molts, and reaches the second larval instar. Then it eats very much, and it molts to its third in star. When the larvae are fully grown it becomes restless and begins to wander. It is now in its prepupal stage.

The prepupae then molts into apupae, but keeps the third larval instars skin, which become the so called pupariurn. Typically it takes between one week and two weeks from the egg to, the pupae stage. The exact time depends on the species and the temperature in the surroundings.

The theory behind estimating time of death, or rather the post mortem interval (PMI for short) with the help of insects are very simple, i.e., since insects arrive on the body soon after death, estimating the age of the insects will also lead to an estimation of the time of death.

To Know-Body Removal at the Scene of Death

After death, a succession of fungi, bacteria and animals will colonize the dead body. The substrate on which the body is lying will also change over time. Leakage of fluids from the dead body will lead to the disappearance of-certain insects, and other. insects will increase as the time goes. A forensic entomologist can then look for how long the body has been there by looking at the fauna at the body, and also estimate the time the body has been lying there by sampling soil insects underneath the dead body.

If there is a difference in the estimates, and the analysis of the soil suggests a short PMI, and the analysis of the body fauna suggests a longer PMI, one can suspect that the body has beenmoved; One can also see that a body has been lying at a particular place long time after the body has been removed, both by botanical means, and by analysis of the soil fauna.

Sometimes dead bodies are found in concealed environments, where blowûies have no access. If there are blowflies, it means that the body has been moved there. Some Calliphorids are heliophilic, that is, they prefer to lay their eggs on warm surfaces; which means that they usually occur where the bodies lies in sunny places.

Other blowflies prefer shade. For example, Lucilia species prefer sunlight, and Calliphora prefer more shady conditions Some species are synanthropic and occurs in urban areas; other species are not synanthropic and occurs in rural areas. Callzphorcr vicina is a synantropic fly, very common in cities and Calliphor a vomiforia is a more rural species, seldom caught in cities.

Analyzing the Scene for Entomological Evidence

To make the most use of entomological evidence at a crime scene, an experienced and Well trained forensic entomologist should do the collecting at the scene. The exact procedure at the crime -scene varies with the type of habitat, but in general the work forensic entomologist can be divided in five parts.

1. Visual observation and notations at the scene.
2. Initiation of climatological data collection at the surrounding places nearby or at the crime scene.
3. Collection of specimens from the body before body removal.
4. Collection of specimen from the surrounding area, i.e., up to 6 mt from the body, before removal of the remains.
5. Collection of specimens from directly under and ill close proximity to the remains within one meter or less, after the body has been removed from the place it was discovered.

Observations of Insects at the Crime Scene

An entomologist will probably observe elements that the investigators will ignore, and vice versa.

Following should be looked for at the crime scene;

1. The type of habitat the crime scene is located in? Is it rural, urban/suburban or aquatic? Is it a forest, a roadside, a closed building, an open building, a pond, a lake, a river, or another habitat types.
2. The type of habitat dictates 'what types' of insects that could be found on the body. Finding of insects typical of other habitats than the crime scene may suggest that the body has been dumped estimate the number and kinds of flying and crawling insects.
3. Locations of major infestations associated with the body and surrounding area. These infestations may be egg, larval pupal or adult stages, alone or in any combinations of the above.
4. Immature stages of particular adult insects observed. These stages can include eggs, larvae, pupae, empty pupal cases, cast larval skins, fecal material, and exit holes or feeding marks on the remains should be noted.
5. Any insect predation such as beetles, ants and wasps or insect parasites.
6. The exact position of the body: compass -direction of the main axis, position of the extremities, position of head and

face, noting of which body parts are in contact with substrate, noting where it would be sunlight and shade during a normal daylight cycle.

7. Note insect activity within 3-6 in of the body. Observe flying, resting or crawling insect adults or larvae or pupae Within this proximity to the body
8. Any unusual naturally occurring, man-made, or scavenger caused phenomenon which could alter the environmental effects on the body, i.e., trauma or mutilation of the body, burning, covering, burial; movement, or dismernberment.

Photographs should be taken of all this conditions present at the crime scene, with close-up photos of the different stages of insect found before collecting.

Climatological Data at the Scene

The length of the insect life cycle is determined mostly by temperature and relative humidity in the environment development takes place. The following climatological data should be collected at the scene:

1. Ambient temperature can be evaluated by taking readings - at 0.3 to 1.3 m heights in close proximity to the body, and ground temperature can be obtained by placing the thermometer on the ground, immediately above any surface ground cover.
2. Body surface temperatures should be obtained by placing the thermometer on the skin surface; under-body interface temperature can be obtained by sliding the thermometer between the body and the ground surface, and maggot mass temperatures can be obtained by inserting the thermometer into the center of the maggot mass.
3. Soil temperatures should be taken immediately after body removal at a ground point which was under the decomposing body. Likewise, it is important to take soil temperatures at a second point 1-2 in away from the body. These temperatures should be taken at 3 levels: Directly under any ground cover, i.e., grass, leaves, etc., at four cm soil depth and at twenty cm soil depth.

4. Weather data for the scene should be collected from the nearest meteorological station. Minimum requirements should be maximum and minimum temperature and amount of precipitation. Any other information is also welcome, and may aid in the reconstruction of the events. The climatological data should extend back to the time the victim was last seen.

Collection of Entomological Specimens

A passive technique for collecting adult insects at the crime scene is by using sticky traps with a slow drying adhesive substance. These traps are made from waxed cardboards with a pup tent configuration set at approximately 60 degree angle with sticky material on both exposed sides. This trap will collect many insects in a few minutes. An insect net can be used to collect flying insects.

Eggs, larvae, pupae and adults of insects on the surface of the human remains should be collected and preserved to show the state of the entomological data at the time of discovery. Insects within the body should not be collected before the autopsy. If there is enough insects, samples of egg, larvae and pupae should be collected alive and placed on a reading medium such as raw beef liver.

Rearing to the adult stage makes identification easier, and may give vital clues to the PMI estimation. It is important that the temperature in the rearing container is as constant as possible, in the range of 20-27 degrees Celsius. It is absolutely necessary that the temperature is recorded in the rearing container.

Conclusion

It is concluded that forensic entomology is very important in the investigation of homicide and other similar cases because this provides an approximate postmortem determination of cadaver such as number of hours after death, cause of death, the possible movement of the corpse after death and or whether contraband played a role in the death of a victim.

The broad field of forensic entomology is commonly broken down into three general areas: medico-legal, urban, and stored product pests. The medico- legal section focuses on the criminal component of the legal system and deals with the necrophagous feeding insects that typically infest human remains. The urban aspect deals with the insects that affect man and his immediate environment.

12

Radiation Poisoning

Radiation is used in medicine, to generate electricity, to make food last longer, to sterilize equipment, for carbon dating of archeological finds, and many other reasons.

Ionizing radiation happens when the atomic nucleus of an unstable atom decays and starts releasing ionizing particles.

When these particles come into contact with organic material, such as human tissue, they will damage them if levels are high enough, in a short period of time. This can lead to burns, problems with the blood, gastrointestinal system, cardiovascular and central nervous system, cancer, and sometimes death.

If an accident happens, for example, the earthquake in Fukushima, Japan, in 2011, or the explosion at Chernobyl, Ukraine in 1986, radiation can become dangerous.

Depending on the dose, the effects of radiation can be lethal.

Radiation poisoning happens when a radioactive substance gives off particles that get into a person's body and cause multiple organ failure.

Radiation dosage can measured in various ways. Some of the units used are Grays, Sieverts, rems, and rads. They are used in a similarway, but 0.1 rad is equivalent to 100 Gray.

Below 30 rads: Mild symptoms will occur in the blood

From 30 to 200 rads: The person may become ill.

From 200 to 1,000 rads: The person may become seriously ill.

Over 1,000 rads: This will be fatal.

According to the Centers for Disease Control and Prevention (CDC), radiation sickness, or acute radiation syndrome (ARS) is diagnosed when:

A person receives over 70 rads from a source outside their body

The dose affects the whole body, or most of it, and is able to penetrate to the internal organs

The dose is received in a short time, usually within minutes

A person who experiences an atomic explosion will receive two doses of radiation, one during the explosion, and another from fallout, when radioactive particles float down after the explosion.

Signs and symptoms

Radiation sickness can be acute, happening soon after exposure, or chronic, where symptoms appear over time or after some time, possibly years later.

The signs and symptoms of acute radiation poisoning are:

vomiting, diarrhea, and nausea

loss of appetite

malaise, or feeling unwell

headache

rapid heartbeat

Symptoms depend on the dose, and whether it is a single dose or repeated.

A dose of as low as 30 rads can lead to:

loss of white blood cells

nausea and vomiting

headaches

A dose of 300 rads dose may result in:

temporary hair loss

damage to nerve cells

damage to the cells that line the digestive tract

Stages of radiation sickness

Symptoms of severe radiation poisoning will normally go through four stages.

Prodomal stage: Nausea, vomiting, and diarrhea, lasting from a few minutes to several days

Latent stage: Symptoms seem to disappear, and the person appears to recover

Overt stage: Depending on the type of exposure, this can involve problems with the cardiovascular, gastrointestinal, hematopoietic, and central nervous system (CNS)

Recovery or death: There may be a slow recovery, or the poisoning will be fatal.

Hematopoietic stem cells, or bone marrow cells, are the cells that all other blood cells derive from.

Different doses, different effects

The risk of illness depends on the dose. Very low doses of radiation are all around us all the time, and they do not have any effect. It also depends on the area of the body that is exposed.

If the whole body is exposed to, say, 1,000 rads within a short time, this could be fatal.

A person who is exposed to 3,000 rads will experience nausea and vomiting, and they may experience confusion and a loss of consciousness within a few hours. Tremors and convulsions will occur 5 to 6 hours after exposure. Within 3 days, there will be coma and death.

People who experience repeated doses, or who appear to recover, may have long-term effects.

These include:

a loss of white blood cells, making it harder for the body to fight infection reduction in platelets, increasing the risk of internal or external bleeding

fertility problems, including loss of menstruation and reduced libido

changes in kidney function, which can lead to anemia, high blood pressure, and other problems within a few months

There may also be skin redness, cataracts, and heart problems.

Localized exposure may lead to changes in the skin, loss of hair, and possibly skin cancer.

Exposure to certain parts of the body is more dangerous than others, for example, the intestines.

The effects of radiation are cumulative. Damage to cells is irreversible.

Sources of radiation

Exposure to radiation can result from workplace exposure or an industrial accident, radiation therapy, or even deliberate poisoning, as in the case of the former Russian spy, Alexander Litvinenko, who was murdered in London by polonium 210 placed in his tea.

The Swiss scientists who tested former Palestinian leader Yasser Arafat 's remains after the exhumation of his body in November 2012 discovered levels of polonium at least 18 times higher than usual in Arafat's ribs, pelvis and in soil that absorbed his bodily fluid, the results "moderately support the proposition that the death was the consequence of poisoning with polonium-210".

CT scans should only be carried out when necessary, as they expose a person to more radiation than is usual in everyday life.

Most people are exposed to an average of around 0.62 rads, or 620 Gray each year.

Half of this comes from radon in the air, from the Earth, and from cosmic rays. The other half comes from medical, commercial, and industrial sources. Spread over a year, this is not significant in terms of health.

Levels of radiation from an x-ray are not high, but they occur at one moment.

A chest x-ray gives the equivalent of 10 days' exposure to radiation

Mammogram gives the equivalent of 7 weeks' normal exposure

PET or CT used as part of nuclear medicine exposes a person to the equivalent of 8 years of radiation

A CT scan of the abdomen and pelvis gives the equivalent of 3 years' normal exposure

Nuclear medicine is used to target the thyroid in people with a thyroid disorder. Other types of medical treatment include radiation therapy for cancer.

Living at a higher altitude, for example, in the plateau of New Mexico and Colorado, increase exposure, as does traveling in an airplane. Radon gas in homes also contributes.

Food, too, contains small amounts of radiation. The food and water we drink is responsible for exposure to around 0.03 rads in a year.

The many activities that can expose people to sources of radiation include:

watching television

flying in an airplane

passing through a security scanner

using a microwave or cell phone

Smokers have a higher exposure than non-smokers, as tobacco contains a substance that can decay to become polonium 210.

Astronauts have the highest exposure of anyone. They may be exposed to 25 rads in one Space Shuttle mission.

Following are the suggested procedure to ascertain the death from radiation;

Toxicological screening

Exhumation procedure

Genetic identification

Radiometric, and statistical tests

Biokinetic calculation procedure

Radioanalytical analysis

Bayesian analysis

13
Medico-legal Sections in IPC, Cr PC, and IEA

Injuries Related

Section 44 IPC:

Definition of Injury

Any harm whatever illegally caused to any person in body, mind, reputation or property.

Section 319 IPC: Hurt

Hurt means bodily pain, disease or infirmity caused to any person.

Section 320 IPC Grievous Injury

Any of the following injuries are grievous.

1. Emasculation (Depriving a male of masculine vigour)
2. Permanent privation of sight of either eye.
3. Permanent privation of the hearing of either ear.
4. Privation of any member or joint (member means an organ or a limb being part of man capable of performing a distinct function).
5. Destruction or permanent impairing of powers of any member or joint.
6. Permanent disfiguration of the head or face.
7. Fracture or dislocation of a bone or tooth.

8. Any hurt which endangers life, or which causes the victim to be in severe bodily pain, or unable to follow his ordinary pursuits for a period of 20 days.

321 IPC: Defines "Voluntarily Causing Hurt"

322 IPC: Defines "Voluntarily Causing Grievous Hurt"

323 IPC: Describes Punishment for Voluntarily Causing Hurt. Shall be imprisonment which may extend for one year with or without fine which may be Rs 1000/-.

324 IPC: Describes Punishment for Voluntarily Causing Hurt by dangerous weapon shall be imprisonment for upto 3 years with or without fine.

325 IPC: Describes Punishment for Voluntarily Causing Grievous Hurt. Shall be imprisonment which may extend for 7 year with or without fine.

326 IPC: Describes Punishment for Voluntarily Causing Grievous Hurt by dangerous weapon or means. Shall be imprisonment for life or for 10 years with or without fine.

327 IPC: Punishment for causing hurt to extort property shall be 10 years with or without fine.

328 IPC: Punishment of causing hurt by means of poison etc. shall be imprisonment upto 10 years with or without fine.

351 IPC: Defines Assault: Threat/attempt to apply force Whoever makes any gesture, or preparation intending or knowing it to be likely that such gesture, or preparation will cause any person present to apprehend that he who makes the gesture or preparation is about to use criminal force to that person, is said to commit an assault.

353 IPC: Punishment for causing assault shall be imprisonment upto 2 years with or without fine.

354 IPC: Punishment for causing assault to women with intend to outrage her modesty shall be imprisonment upto 2 years with or without fine.

498A IPC: Punishment for husband or relative of husband of a women subjecting her to cruelty, shall be imprisonment for upto 3 years with or without fine.

Forensic Psychiatry, Consent and Alcohol

82 IPC: Act of a child under 7 years of age Nothing is an offence which is done by a child under 7 years of age.

83 IPC: Act of child b/w 7-12 years. Nothing is an offence which is done by a child above 7 years and under 12 years, who has not attained maturity of understanding it judge the nature and consequences of his conduct on that occasion.

84 IPC: Insanity

Nothing is an offence which done by a person who at the time of doing it, is by reason of unsoundedness of mind, is incapable of knowing the nature of the act, or that what is doing is wrong or contrary to law of the land. The meaning of insanity in civil law, medicine and neuroscience is different from its meaning in criminal law. It is described in Indian Lunatic Act, 1912.

Insanity in Medical Terms

There is a difference between the medical definitions of insanity. According to medical science, insanity is a disorder of the mind that impairs the mental facilities of a man14. Insanity is another name for mental abnormalities due to various factors and exists in various degrees15. Insanity is popularly denoted by idiocy, madness, lunacy, to describe mental derangement, mental disorder and all other forms of mental abnormalities known to medical science.

Section 85 IPC: Act under intoxication

Nothing is an offence which is done by a person, who at the time of doing it, is by reason of intoxication, incapable of knowing the nature of the actor that he is doing what is either wrong or contrary to law; provided the thing which intoxicated him was administered to him without his knowledge or against his will.

Section 86 IPC:

In cases where an act done is not an offence unless done with a particular knowledge or intent, a person who does the act in a state of intoxication shall be liable to be dealt wit has if he had the some knowledge as he would have if he had not been intoxicated, unless the thing which intoxicated him was administered to him without his knowledge or against his will.

Thus, drunkenness caused by voluntary use of alcohol or some other intoxicating drug is no excuse for the commission of a crime but insanity produced by drunkenness, voluntary or otherwise, absolves one from criminal responsibility if it can stand the usual legal tests applied in other forms of insanity.

87 IPC: Consent above 18 years to suffer harm a person below 18 years of age cannot give a valid consent, whether express or implied to suffer any harm which may result from an act not intended or not known to cause death or grievous hurt.

88 IPC: Consent above 18 years

A person can give valid consent to suffer any harm which may result from an act, not intended or not known to cause death, done in good faith and forits benefit

89 IPC: Consent below 12 years

A child below 12 years of age and an insane person cannot give valid consent to suffer any harm which may result from an act done in good faith and for its benefit.

90 IPC: Consent under fear

A consent given by a person under fear of injury, or due to misunderstanding of a fact is not valid

Section 53(i) CrPC:

An accused may be examined by a medical practitioner at the request of a police officer using reasonably necessary force.

Section 53 (ii) Cr P: 1973- Medical Evidence

Whenever the person of a female accused is to be examined, the examination shall be made only by orunder the supervision of a female registered medical practitioner.

A medical man is required to provide assistance to the cause of justice by furnishing certificates and reports consequent upon examination of a living person and a dead.

1. In civil cases, the opinion of a medical expert is relevant to prove,

i. Age, in matters of minority and majority disputes,

ii. Death, whether natural or unnatural,

iii. Ill health, required for leave on medical grounds from offices and exemption from court attendance,

iv. Certificate of fitness for Govt. Services and other jobs, whatever this is required according to rules,

v. Mental conditions of a person at the time of making a will,

vi. Mental capabilities of a person to manage his own state of affairs,

2. In criminal matters, the opinion of a medical expert may be required to prove;

i. Types of hurt, injuries and their severity,

ii. Post-mortem report regarding the cause of death, time since death, manner of death, type of weapon or to prove the actual weapon involved in the case,

iii. Insanity and other mental disorders,

iv. Age, to decide minority or majority in sexual assault cases, validity of marriage and cases of kidnapping,

v. Drunkenness, delirium tremens, etc,

vi. Virginity or otherwise of a woman,

vii. Impotence, sterility of a man,

viii. Pregnancy and childbirth, gestation period,

ix. Medico- legal facts in sexual offences,

x. Dying declaration

Section 54 CrPC:

An arrested person may be examined at his request by a medical practitioner to detect evidence in his favour.

Injury: Murder and Culpable Homicide

Section 299 IPC: Defines Culpable Homicide

Whoever causing death by doing an act with the intention of causing death, or with the intention of causing such bodily injury as so likely to cause death, or with the knowledge that he is likely by such act to cause death, commits the offence of culpable homicide.

Section 300 IPC: Murder

Culpable homicide is murder:

If the act by which the death is caused is done with the intention of causing death or, If it is done with the intention of causing such bodily injury as the offender knows to be likely to cause death or, If it is done with the intention of causing such bodily injury which is sufficient in the ordinary course of nature to cause death or,

If the person committing the act knows that it is so imminently dangerous, that it must in all probability cause death or such bodily injury as is likely to cause death and commits such act without any excuse.

Culpable homicide is not murder:

a. If the offender whilst deprived of the power of self control by grave and sudden provocation causes the death of the person who gave the provocation, or causes the death of other person by mistake or accident.

b. If in good faith of the right of private defence of person Or property, the offender exceeds the power given to him bylaw and causes the death of the person against whom he is exercising such right of defence, without premeditation and without any intention of doing more harm than what is necessary- for the purpose of such defence.

c. If the offender, being a public servant or aiding a public servant acting for the advancement of public justice, exceeds the powers given to him by law and causes death by doing an act which he, in good faith believes to be lawful and necessary for the due discharge of his duty and without any ill-will towards the person whose death is caused.

d. If the act is committed without premeditation in a sudden fight in the heat of passion or a sudden quarrel, without the offender having taken any undue advantage or acting in a cruel or unusual manner. (It is immaterial which party offers the provocation or commits the first assault.)

e. When the person whose death is caused, being above the age of 18 years, suffers death or takes the risk of death with his own consent.

301 IPC: Culpable homicide by causing death of a person other than whose death is intended.

Section 302 IPC: Punishment for murder

Whoever commits murder, shall be punished with death or transportation for life and shall also be liable to fine.

303 IPC: Punishment for murder by a life convict.

Section 304 IPC: Punishment for culpable homicide not amounting to murder. Whoever commits culpable homicide not amounting to murder,

1. shall be punished with imprisonment for life or imprisonment of either description for a term which may extend to 10 years and shall also be liable to fine, if the act by which death is caused is done with the intention of causing death or of causing such bodily injury as is likely to cause death.

or

2. with imprisonment of either description which may extend to 10 years or with fine or both if the act by which death is caused is done with the knowledge that it is likely to cause death but without any intention to cause death or to cause such bodily injury as is likely to cause death,

Section 304 A IPC: Causing death by negligence

Whoever, causes the death of a person by doing any rash or negligent act riot amounting to culpable homicide shall be punished with imprisonment of either description for a term which may extend to 2 years, or with fine or with both,

304 B IPC: Dowry Death

when death of a women occurs due to burn or other bodily injury or in circumstances other than normal, within 7 years of marriage, and it is seen that she was subjected to cruelty or harassment by her husband or any relative of her husband for or in connection with the demand of dowry, such death shall be called dowry death and the husband or his relative shall be deemed to have caused her death.

305 IPC: Punishment of abetement of suicide of a child under 18 years of age or an insane shall be upto 10 years with or without fine.

Section 306 IPC: Punishment for abetment of suicide Imprisonment of either description for a term which may extend to 10 years and fine.

Section 307 IPC: Punishment for attempt to murder Imprisonment of either description for a term upto 10 years and fine.

Section 309 IPC: Attempt to commit suicide

Punished with imprisonment for 1 year or with fine or with both.

Simple Injuries: All injuries which are not grievous are simple.

Dangerous Injuries: Dangerous injuries are those which cause imminent danger to life, either by involvement of important organs or structures, or extensive area of the body. If no surgical aid is available, such injuries may prove fatal.

Sexual Offences and Criminal Abortion

It is the induced destruction and expulsion of the foetus from the mother's womb unlawfully. In other words, it is abortion not in accordance with the provisions of the MfP Act, 1971. It is generally induced between the second and third months of pregnancy and occasionally between the fourth and fifth months.

Legal bearing

Sections 312, 313, 314, 315 and *316 IPC* refer to the offence of criminal miscarriage and punishment a warded for these offences.

Section 312 IPC: Causing miscarriage

Whoever voluntarily causes a woman with child to miscarry, shall if such miscarriage be not caused in good faith for the purpose of saving the life of the woman, be punished with imprisonment of either description for a term which may extend to 3 years, or with fine, or with both; and if the woman be quick with the child, shall be punished with imprisonment of either description for a term which may extend to 7 years and shall also be liable to fine.

Section 313 IPC: Causing miscarriage without woman's consent

Whoever voluntarily causes a woman with child to miscarry without the consent of the woman, whether the woman is quick with the child or not, shall be punished with transportation for life or with imprisonment of either description for a term which may extend to 10 years and shall also be liable to fine.

Section 314 IPC: Death caused by an act done with intent to cause miscarriage

Whoever with intent to cause miscarriage of a woman with child, does any act which causes the death of the woman, shall be punished with imprisonment of either description for a term which may extend to 10 years and shall also be liable to fine; and if the act is done without the consent of the woman, shall be punished with either transportation for life or with the above mentioned punishment. Explanation: It is not necessary for the offender to know that the act is likely to cause death.

Section 315 IPC: Act done with intent to prevent child being born alive or to cause it to die after birth.

Whoever before the birth of any child, does any act with the intention of preventing that child from being born alive or causing it to die after its birth and does by such an act prevent that child from being born alive or causes it to die after its birth shall be punished with imprisonment of either description for a term.

Which may extend to 10 years or with fine or with both, provided the act is not done in good faith for the purpose of saving the life of the mother.

Section 316 IPC: Causing death of quick unborn child by act amounting to culpable homicide

A person would be guilty of culpable homicide if he caused the death of a pregnant woman by an act which he knew was likely to cause her death. If his act injured the woman and did not cause her death, but caused the death of her unborn quick child, he would be guilty of the offence defined under this section and shall be punished with imprisonment for a term which may extend to 10 years and shall also be liable to fine.

Section 375 IPC: Definition of Rape

Unlawful sexual intercourse by a man,

a. with his own wife under the age of 15 years or,
b. with any other woman under the age of 16 years, with or without her consent or,
c. with any other woman above the age of 16 years, against her will, without her consentor,
d. with her consent, when her consent has been obtained by putting her or any person in whom she is interested in fear of death or hurtor,
e. with her consent, when the man, knows that he is not her husband and that her consent is given because she believes that he is another man to whom she is or believes herself to be lawfully married or,
f. with her consent, when at the time of giving such consent, by reason of unsoundness of mind, or intoxication, or the administration of any stupefying or unwholesome substance, she is unable to understand the nature and consequences of that to which she gives consent.

Section 376 IPC: Punishment for Rape

Whoever commits rape, shall be punished with imprisonment of either description for a term which shall not be less than 7 years but which maybe for life, or for a term which may extend to 10 years and shall also beliable to fine.

Custodial rape

Rape by police officer or public servant who abuses his position of authority is punishable by imprisonment for at least 10 years to life and fine.

Section 376A IPC: Marital rape

Whoever has sexual intercourse with his own wife, who is living separately from him under a degree of separation or under any custom or usage without her consent, shall be punished with imprisonment of either description for a term which may extend to 2 years and shall also be liable to fine.

Section 376B IPC:

Sexual intercourse not-amounting to rape by a public servant who induces or seduces a woman in his custody to have sexual intercourse with him shall be punishable with imprisonment of upto 5 years and fine.

Section 376C IPC:

Sexual intercourse not amounting to rape by a superintendent of jail, remand home or other places of custody who induces or

seduces any female inmate to have sexual intercourse with him shall be punishable with imprisonment of upto 5 years and fine.

Section 376D IPC:

Sexual intercourse not amounting to rape by a member of the management or staff of a hospital who taking advantage of his position induces or seduces any woman in the hospital to have sexual intercourse with him shall be punishable with imprisonment of upto 5 years and fine.

Section 114A IEA:

In a prosecution for rape, where the question is whether sexual intercourse was without the consent of the woman, and she states in her evidence that she did not consent, the court shall presume that she did not consent.

Section 228A IPC:

Disclosure of identity of the victim against whom an offence under sections 376, 37 6A-D IPC is alleged to have been committed, is not permitted except by due authorization. Any person who prints or publishes without authorization by a proper authority the name or any material which will result in identifying the victim of rape shall be punished with imprisonment of upto 2 years and fine.

Section 354 IPC: Indecent assault

Indecent assault on a female committed with intent or knowledge to outrage her modesty is punishable with imprisonment of either description for a term which may extend to 2 years or fine or with both.

Section 377 IPC: Unnatural offences

Whoever, voluntarily has carnal intercourse against the order of nature with any man, woman or animal shall be punished with transportation for life or with imprisonment of either description for a term which mayextend to 10 years and shall also be liable to fine.

Poisoning

Section 272 IPC: Punishment for adulterating food or drink intended for sale, so as to make the same noxious, may extend upto 6 months imprisonment of either term and/or fine upto one thousand rupees.

Section 273 IPC: Punishment for selling noxious food or drink may be imprisonment of either description for a period of 6 months and or fine upto one thousand rupees.

Section 274 IPC: Punishment for adulteration of drugs in any form with any change in its effect knowing that it will be sold and used as un-adulterated drug, may be imprisonment of either description for a period of 6 months and or fine.

Section 275 IPC: Punishment for knowingly selling adulterated drugs with less efficacy or altered action serving it for use as unadulterated may be imprisonment of either description for 6 months and or fine.

Section 276 IPC: Punishment for selling a drug as a different drug or Preparation may be imprisonment of either description which may extend upto 6 months and or fine.

Note: In the State of West Bengal, the punishment for these offences described under sections 272 to 276 may be upto imprisonment for life with or without fine.

Section 277 IPC: Punishment for fouling water of public spring or reservoir may be imprisonment of either description which may extend up to a period of 3 months and or fine.

Section 278 IPC: Punishment for voluntarily making atmosphere noxious to health is fine which may extend upto five hundred rupees.

Section 284 IPC: Punishment for negligent conduct with respect to poisonous substance may be imprisonment of either description which may extend upto 6 months and or fine which may extend upto one thousand rupees.

Section 328 IPC: Punishment for causing hurt by means of poison or any stupefying, intoxicating or unwholesome drug or any other thing with the intent to commit an offence shall be imprisonment of either description for a term which may extend to ten years with or without fine.

Part II
Toxicology

14

Introduction to Toxicology

During the past decades industrialization and agricultural development, paralleled with increased health care have changed life in various ways. Average life expectancy rose, due to better control of epidemics and infectious diseases. However, increased industrialization and agricultural development were the chief cause of pollution that had profound influences on our lives. Man, the other animals, & the plants in the modern world are increasingly being exposed to chemicals of an enormous variety. Nearly everyone is at risk of toxic exposures to hazardous substances in the ambient environment. In recent years, awareness of the problem of human & animal exposure to potentially toxic chemicals in our environment has grown. So toxicology has a very important role to play in modern society & consequently it is now growing rapidly as a new subject. This short chapter presents an overview of the broad topic of toxicology.

Definition of Toxicology

The word toxicology is derived from two Greek words; toxikon, meaning poisonous substance into which arrow heads were dipped and logos, meaning study.

Toxicology is the qualitative and quantitative study of the adverse or toxic effect of chemicals and other anthropogenic materials or xenobiotics on organisms. It also deals with food and cosmetics for public consumption both in alive or dead victims.

It is the science of poison & its scope has been enlarging. It is one of the multidisciplinary fields of science.

It has got another dimension: the social, the moral & legal aspects of exposure of populations to chemicals of unknown or uncertain hazard.

Historical aspects of toxicology – it is only recently that the study of poisons becomes truly scientific & in the past it was mainly a practical art utilized by murderers & assassins. Poison has played an important part in human history.

In Ancient time (1500 BC) earliest collection of medical records contains many references and recipes for poisons. Dioscorides (50 AD) a Greek physician, classify poisons as animal, plant or mineral & recognized the value of emetics Maimmonides (1135-1204 AD), wrote about poisons and their antidote.

Paracelsus (1493 AD), viewed a poison in the body would be cured by a similar poison but the dosage is very important. Paracelsus summarized his concept in the following famous phrase "All substances are poisons; there is none that is not a poison. The right dose differentiates a poison from a remedy".

Orifila (1787-1853 AD), Spanish physician who contributed to forensic toxicology by devising means of detecting poisonous substances. From then on toxicology began in a more scientific manner & began to include the study of the mechanism of action of poisons.

In the 20th century, toxicology has now become much more than the use of poisons. There are marked improvements in toxicological diagnosis (that ranges from screening to confirmatory tests), & management (production of antidote for them).

Epidemiology

The following toxicological data are derived from American association of poison control center. So it is mostly a description of the epidemiology of unintentional poisoning. It is very difficult to find the primary data of poisoning in our country because most of the screening & confirmatory tests are not done routinely in our set up. Additionally, we don't have well organized poison control center.

Today, poisoning (both accidental and intentional), is a significant contributor to mortality and morbidity. It has been estimated that 7% of all emergency room visits are the result of toxic exposures. Household cleaner, over-the-counter and prescription drugs, cosmetics, and solvents comprise the most frequent human toxic exposures. Young children and elderly are most likely to be accidentally exposed to drugs or household chemicals at home. During adolescence and young adulthood the exposures are more likely to be intentional, either through suicide attempts or experimentation with drugs or alcohol. More than 72.4% of all poison exposures occur in children and adolescents less than 17 years of age. Exposures are equally reported in males and females. However, adult men have been reported to be more at risk of occupational exposures than adult woman. Route of entry of exposures reported was by mouth in most cases: 77% were the result of ingestion, 7.0% were transdermal, 5.9% were ophthalmic; and 5.5% were by inhalation. Site of exposure was a residence in 91.9% of all, followed by the workplace, schools and health facilities. Most poison exposures do not result in clinical toxicity. In general, nearly everyone is at risk of acute and chronic toxic exposures to hazardous substances in the ambient environment.

Toxicologic Terms and Definitions

A. Important toxicologic terms

Toxin: a poison of natural origin.

Poison (Toxicant): a chemical that may harm or kill an organism

Toxicity: is the ability of a chemical agent to cause injury.

It is a qualitative term which depends on the amount of chemical absorbed, severity of the exposure, dose & others. It can be acute (toxic event which occurs soon after acute or limited exposure), or chronic (apply to an event which occurs many weeks, months or years after exposure).

Hazard: is the likelihood that injury will occur in a given situation or setting: the conditions of use and exposure are primary considerations.

Risk: is defined as the expected frequency of the occurrence of an undesirable effect arising from exposure to a chemical or physical agent.

Acute exposure is a single exposure – or multiple exposures occurring over 1 or 2 days.

Chronic exposure is multiple exposures continuing over a longer period of time.

B. Presence of mixtures

Humans normally come in contact with several (or many) different chemicals concurrently or sequentially. The resulting biologic effect of combined exposure to several agents can be characterized as synergistic, additive, Potentiation & antagonistic Synergism-when the effect of two chemicals is greater than the effect of individual chemicals e.g. carbontetrachloride + alcohol= more toxic to the liver than the sum of the individual drugs Additive effect- when the total pharmacological action of two or more chemicals taken together is equivalent to the summation of their individual pharmacological action.

Potentiation effect: the capacity of a chemical to increase the effect of another chemical without having the effect e.g. Disulfiram at non-toxic doses potentiate the toxicity of alcohol & used in the treatment of alcohol abuse.

Antagonism: is the phenomenon of opposing actions of two chemicals on the same system e.g. paracetamol causes serious liver damage when given with alcohol or barbiturates, both of which induce drug metabolizing enzymes.

Basic Classification of Toxicology

Toxicology is broadly divided into different classes depending on research methodology, socio-medical & organ/specific effects.

I. Based on research methodology

A. Descriptive toxicology

Descriptive toxicology deals with toxicity tests on chemicals exposed to human beings and environment as a whole.

B. Mechanistic toxicology

Mechanistic toxicology deals with the mechanism of toxic effects of chemicals on living organisms. This is important for rational treatment of the manifestations of toxicity (e.g. organophosphate poisoning reversed by oximes),prediction of risks (e.g. -organophosphate poisoning '!leads to accumulation of acetylcholine '! activate muscarinic and nicotinic receptors'!respiratory failure) & facilitation of search for safer drugs (e.g. Instead of organophosphates, drugs which reversibly bind to cholinesterase would be preferable in therapeutics)

C. Regulatory toxicology

Regulatory toxicology studies whether the chemical substances has low risk to be used in living systems. e .g. - Food and drug administration regulates drugs, food, cosmetics medical devices &supplies in USA/ European Countries.

- Environmental protection agency regulates pesticides, toxic chemicals, hazardous wastes and toxic pollutants in USA/ European Countries.
- Occupational safety and health administration regulates the safe conditions for employees in USA/ European Countries.
- Public Health & Drugs administration Deptt. - regulates drugs, cosmetics and medical devices & supplies in India.

D. Predictive toxicology

Predictive toxicology studies about the potential and actual risks of chemicals or drugs. This is important for licensing a new drug or chemical for use.

II. Based on specific socio-medical issues

A. Occupational toxicology

Occupational toxicology Deals with chemical found in the workplace e.g., industrial workers may be exposed to these agents during the synthesis, manufacturing or packaging of substances.

Agricultural workers may be exposed to harmful amounts of pesticides during the application in the field.

B. Environmental toxicology

Environmental toxicology deals with the potentially deleterious impact of chemicals, present as pollutants of the environment, to living organisms. Ecotoxicology has evolved as an extension of environmental toxicology. It is concerned with the toxic effects of chemical and physical agents on living organisms, especially in populations and communities with defined ecosystems.

C. Clinical toxicology

Clinical toxicology deals with diagnosis and treatment of the normal diseases or effects caused by toxic substances of exogenous origin i.e., xenobiotics.

D. Forensic toxicology

Forensic toxicology closely related to clinical toxicology. It deals with the medical and legal aspects of the harmful effects of chemicals on man, often in post mortem material, for instance, where there is a suspicion of murder, attempted murder or suicide by poisoning.

III. Based on the organ/system effect

1. Cardiovascular toxicology
2. Renal toxicology
3. Central nervous system toxicology
4. Gastrointestinal toxicology
5. Respiratory toxicology, etc.

IV. Toxicokinetics and Toxicodynamics;

- Toxicokinetics deals with absorption, distribution, biotransformation (biotransformation) and excretion of chemicals.
- Toxicodynamics deals with the biochemical and physiological effects of chemicals to the body and mechanisms of their actions.

A. Toxicokinetics

i. Absorption

Absorption is the process by which the chemical enters the body. It depends on the route of administration, dissociation (to become ionized), dissolution (ability of solid dosage form to become soluble), concentration, blood flow to the site, and the area of the absorptive site.

The common sites of absorption (routes of exposure) are;

Oral route - the GIT is the most important route of absorption, as most acute poisonings involve ingestions.

Dermal route - lipid solubility of a substance is an important factor affecting the degree of absorption through the skin.

Inhalational route - toxic fumes, particulate and noxious gases may be absorbed through the lungs.

Bioavailability is the fraction of unchanged drug reaching the systemic circulation following of non-vascular administration.

Therefore, a portion of the chemical fails to reach the systemic circulation in original form after oral administration.

ii. Distribution

Distribution-is defined as the apparent volume into which a substance is distributed. Volume of distribution (Vd) is calculated from the dose taken and the resulting plasma concentration:

Vd = dose /plasma concentration

The importance of volume of distribution in toxicology is

- Predicting peak blood concentration of the chemical taken
- Calculating the amount of substance in the body to verify the quantity ingested.
- Deciding whether to apply systemic toxin elimination techniques.

Factors determining the rate of distribution of chemicals in the body are

- Protein binding chemicals highly bound to protein have small volume of distribution.
- Plasma concentration – when the volume of distribution of chemicals is small, most of the chemical remains in the plasma
- Physiological barriers – chemicals will not uniformly distributed to the body due to specialized barriers e.g. blood brain barrier
- Affinity of chemicals to certain tissues – the concentration of a chemical in certain tissues after a single dose may persist even when its plasma concentration is reduced e.g. Lead concentrate in bone tissue e.g. A 60 Kg epileptic victim attempted suicide by ingesting Phenytoin tablets. Vd listed is 0.6 L/Kg. Peak blood concentration measured by the laboratory is 50mg/ L. What is the dose of the drug that was taken by the victim?

  Dose=plasma concentration x Vd

  =50mg/L x (0.6L/Kg x 60Kg)

  = 1800mg

iii. Biotransformation (metabolism)

Biotransformation is the biochemical transformation of a chemical. It is a process by which the body transforms a chemical and makes it more water soluble so the chemical can be eliminated more rapidly via the kidney into the urine. Biotransformation can produce metabolites that are pharmacologically active and toxic E.g. parathion'! parathoxon (toxic metabolite). Liver is the major site of biotransformation for many chemicals & other organs that are involved are lungs, kidneys, skin &so on. Interactions during bio-transformation includes two phases of bio-transformation.

Phase I – the drug is converted into more polar compound e.g. oxidation, reduction, & hydrolysis

Phase II (conjugation) – a drug or its metabolite is conjugated with an endogenous substance e.g. glucuronide conjugate

Enzyme inhibition- by this the biotransformation of drugs is delayed & is a cause of increased toxicity

Enzyme induction- by this the bio-transformation of drugs is accelerated & is a cause of therapeutic failure.

First – pass effect – is the bio-transformation of some chemicals by the liver during the initial pass from the portal circulation after oral administration.

Half-life (t ½) -is the time required to reduce the blood concentration of the chemical to half.

IV. Excretion

Excretion is the final means of chemical elimination, either as metabolites or unchanged parent chemical. Excretion through the lungs is the major route for gaseous substances; and in the case of non-volatile water – soluble drugs, the kidneys are the most important routes of excretion. Additional routes include sweat, saliva, tears, nasal secretions, milk, bile and feces. Clearance – elimination of chemicals from the body may be described by the term clearance (CL). It is a quantitative measure of the volume of blood cleared of drug per unit time, usually expressed in milliliter per minute.

Clearance is calculated as follows;

$CL = 0.7\,(VD)/\,(t1/2) = ml/min$

Where the VD is expressed in milliliter per kilogram & the half-life is expressed in minutes or hours.

N.B. - Certain points regarding the toxicokinetics of toxic agents;

Drug absorption after a toxic ingestion may be delayed and prolonged;

The half-life and total body clearance are often lengthened;

Liver-metabolizing enzymes may become saturated, slowing hepatic elimination;

Chemicals with large volumes of distribution are often highly tissue-bound and measures to enhance their elimination are not effective;

Poor perfusion of the liver and kidneys secondary to the toxic effects of the substance may slow clearance.

B. Toxicodynamics

Toxicodynamics is the mechanism of action of a toxic chemical to the body (what chemicals do to the body). The targets for the toxicodynamic actions of toxic chemicals are; Enzymes

Membrane receptors o Intracellular receptors o Ion channel

Toxic effects generally result from adverse cellular, biochemical, or macromolecular changes which attained by; Damage to an enzyme system o Disruption of protein synthesis

DNA damage

Modification of an essential biochemical function

The general dose-response principles are of crucial importance in determining the severity of the intoxication. We have two types of responses so called Quantal dose response (all- or – none response) & graded dose response (when dose increases, the response increases in graded fashion). Both responses show a typical dose response relation (see below). The parameters that are derived from the dose response relationships are Median lethal dose (LD50) – is the dose which is expected to kill 50% of the population in the particular group.

Median effective dose (ED50) –is the dose that produces a desired response in 50% of the test population when pharmacological effects are plotted against dosage.

Median toxic dose (TD50) – is the dose which is expected to bring toxic effect in 50% of the population in the particular group.

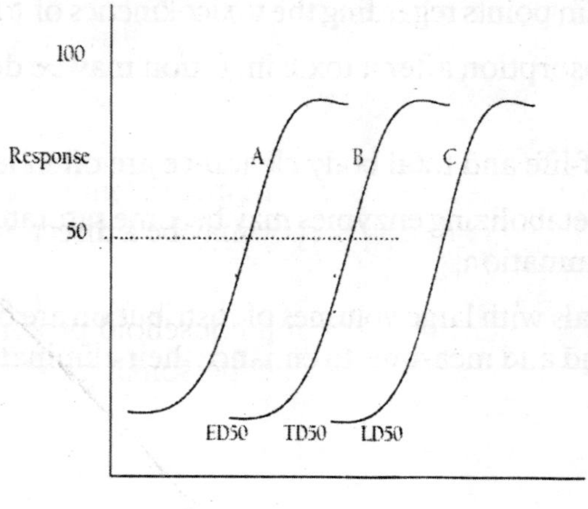

Fig. Comparison of dose–response curves for efficacy (A), toxicity (B), & lethality (C). The effective, toxic, &lethal dosage for 50% of the population in the groupcan be estimated as shown.

Common effects of chemicals to cause symptoms

Chemicals can cause symptoms through the following mechanisms:

a. Interfere with the transport or tissue utilization of oxygen (carbon monoxide, cyanide), resulting in hypoxia or a decrease in an essential substrate such as glucose.

b. Depress or stimulate the CNS, producing coma (sedative-hypnotics) or convulsions (Sympathomimetics such as cocaine, amphetamines)

c. Affect the autonomic nervous system, producing cholinergic action (organophosphate insecticide)

d. Affect the lungs by aspiration (hydrocarbon)

e. Affect the heart and vasculature producing myocardial dysfunction, dysrrhythmias (antiarrhythmic agents) and hypertension or hypotension

f. Produce local damage (caustics and corrosives)

g. Delayed effects on the liver (acetaminophen) or kidneys (heavy metals).

Potential Sources of Toxicities

The potential causes of toxicities include;

Therapeutic agents –drug toxicity can be due to over doses, unusual adverse effects, frequent administrations of therapeutic doses & drug interactions.

Industrial chemicals- these chemicals may contribute to environmental pollution & they may be a direct hazard in the work place they are used.

House-hold chemicals – The top household products ingested are cleaning agents, cosmetics & personal products & berries.

Environmental contaminants- main sources of pollution to the environment are industrial processes, pesticides & smokes from factories & vehicles. Environmental pollutants may be released into the air, water, or dumped onto land.

Natural toxicants- many plants & animals produce toxic substances for both defense & offensive purposes. Natural toxins may feature in poisoning via containing in food, by accidental ingestions of poisonous plants or animals & by stinging & biting

Food additives – have usually low biological activity.

Many different additives are added to food to alter the flavor or colour, prevent spoilage or in some other way change the nature of the food stuff. There are also many potentially toxic substances which are regarded as contaminants.

Traditional medicines (Botanicals) – the medical use of botanicals in their natural &unprocessed form undoubtedly noticed long time ago. The use of botanicals has increased dramatically. Unfortunately, misconceptions regarding safety &efficacy of the agents are common. In fact, these products can be adulterated, misbranded or contaminated. Furthermore, the doses for active botanical substances may be higher. Adverse effects have been documented for a variety of botanical medications.

Drugs of abuse - Excessive or improper use of drugs or other substances for non-medical purposes, usually for altering consciousness but also for body building is known as abuse of drug. There are a lot of drugs of abuse with high potential of dependence & tolerance (e.g., alcohol, nicotine, etc.)

Environmental Considerations

Certain chemical and physical characteristics are known to be important for estimating the potential hazard involved for environmental toxicants. In addition to information regarding effects on different organisms, knowledge about the following properties is essential to predict the environmental impact:

The degradability of the substance; its mobility through air, water and soil; whether or not bio-accumulation occurs; and its transport and bio-magnification through food chains.

If the intake of a long-lasting contaminant by an organism exceeds the latter's ability to metabolize or excrete the substance, the chemical accumulates within the tissues of the organism (e.g., DDT). This is called bio-accumulation.

Although the concentration of a contaminant may be virtually undetectable in water, it may be magnified hundred or thousand time as the contaminant passes up the food chain. This is called bio-magnification.

Chemicals that are poorly degraded (by abiotic or biotic pathways) exhibits environmental persistence and thus can accumulate. Lipophilic substances tend to accumulate in body fat, resulting in tissue residues. When the toxicant is incorporated in to the food chain, bio-magnification occurs as one species feed upon others and concentrates the chemical. The pollutants that have the widest environmental impact are poorly degradable & relatively mobile in air, water and soil, exhibits bio-accumulation; and also exhibits bio-magnification.

In eco-toxicology there are three interacting components; the toxicant, the environment and the organisms (community, population or ecosystem).

Poison Prevention & Control Strategies

a. Keep all household poisons separate from food.

b. Keep all products in their original containers.

c. Always read all labels carefully before using the product.

d. Never give or take any medication in the dark.

e. Dispose all products in a safe and proper manner.

f. Encourage periodic home hunts and dispose of old medicine.

g. Teach children never to take medication unless given by an adult they know and trust.

h. Buy only those drugs supplied in childproof packaging.

i. Once a child has been poisoned, be on the alert for repeat episodes.

j. Teach children not eat plants or berries.

k. Store all drugs or potentially toxic substances out of sight and out of reach of children: use cabinet locks.

15
General Approach to A Victim of Poison

Diagnosis of poisoning may be difficult. The victim may either be unconscious or may not admit self-poisoning. Therefore, a suspicious mind is required. When acute poisoning is suspected, the clinician needs to ask a number of questions in order to establish a diagnosis (history of present illness). In the case of an unconscious (comatose) victim, the circumstances in which the victim was found and whether any tablet, bottles or other containers (scene residues) were present can be important. If the victim is awake, he or she should be questioned about the presence of poisons in the home or workplace. The victim's past medical history (including drugs prescribed and any psychiatric illness), occupation and hobbies may also be relevant, since they may indicate possible access to specific poisons.

Physical examination of the victim may indicate; The poison or class of poison involved.

The clinical features associated with some common poisons may be specific. For example, the combination of pin-point pupils, hyper salivation, incontinence and respiratory depression suggests poisoning with a cholinesterase inhibitor such as an organophosphorus pesticide. However, the value of this approach is limited, if a number of poisons with different actions have been absorbed. Moreover, many drugs have similar effects on the body, while some clinical features may be the result of secondary effects such as anoxia. Thus, if a victim is admitted with depressed respiration and pin-point pupils, this strongly suggests poisoning with an opioid.

Diagnoses other than poisoning must also be considered, for example, coma can be caused by a cerebrovascular accident, uncontrolled diabetes infections as well as poisoning. The availability of the results of urgent biochemical and hematological tests is obviously important in these circumstances.

Finally, poisoning with certain compounds may be misdiagnosed, especially if the victim presents in the later stages of the episode. Examples include: c a r d i o r e s p i r a t o r y a r r e s t (cyanide), h e p a t i t i s (paracetamol) and so on.

N.B. Generally Physical examination should include:

Vital signs

Evaluation of specific parts of the body

Investigations

a. *General laboratory tests*

Hematological

Biochemical

b. Toxicological studies

c. Electrocardiogram

d. X-ray findings

Principles of Management of Poisoning

The initial management of a patient with altered mental status follows the follow the same approach regardless of the poison involved. The airway should be checked, breathing &circulation should be assessed. Then symptomatic &supportive measures are taken. After this, one can begin in a more detailed evaluation to make a specific diagnosis. Therefore, in principle, during poisoning, one should treat the victim first followed by treating the poison itself.

General measures

1. Supportive measures

The first priority is to establish & maintain vital functions. Subsequently, most victims can be treated successfully using supportive care alone.

- Maintain airway, adequate ventilation & oxygenation, provide tracheal intubation if required.
- If comatose, administer glucose, thiamine, & oxygen
- For seizures, administer anticonvulsants

2. *Principles of toxin eliminations*

- If the poison has been inhaled, the victim should first be removed from the contaminated environment.
- If skin contamination has occurred, contaminated clothing should be removed and the skin washed with an appropriate fluid, usually water.
- In adult victims, gastric aspiration and lavage (stomach washout) are often performed, if the poison has been ingested, to minimize the risk of continued absorption.
- Similarly, in children emesis can be induced by the oral administration of syrup of ipecacuanha (ipecac).
- The absorption of any residue remaining after gastric lavage can be minimized by leaving a high dose of activated charcoal in the stomach.
- The role of lavage and induced emesis in preventing absorption is currently being examined, as is the effectiveness of a single dose of activated charcoal. However, repeated oral administration of activated charcoal appears to be effective in enhancing elimination of certain poisons.
- Specific therapeutic procedures, such as antidotal and active elimination therapy are sometimes indicated. The results of either a qualitative or a quantitative toxicological analysis may be required before some treatments are commenced because they are not without risk to the victim. In general, specific therapy is only started when the nature and/or the amount of the poison(s) involved are known. Antidotes or protective agents are only available for a limited number of

poisons. In summery there are four main methods of enhancing elimination of the poison from the systemic circulation:

1. Repeated oral activated charcoal;
2. Forced diuresis with alteration of urine pH;
3. Peritoneal dialysis and haemodialysis; and
4. Haemoperfusion.

Some antidotes &protective agents used to treat acute poisoning;

Antidote Indication

Acetylcysteine Paracetamol

Atropine Organophosphate

Deferoxamine Iron

Methylene blue Nitrates

Physiostigmine Atropine

Naloxone Opioids

Pyridoxine Isoniazid

16

Clinical Toxicology Laboratory

Clinical toxicology involves the detection and treatment of poisonings caused by a wide variety of substances, including household and industrial products, animal poisons and venoms, environmental agents, pharmaceuticals, and illegal drugs. The toxicology laboratory must provide appropriate testing in three general areas: Identification of agents responsible for acute or chronic poisoning; Detection of drugs of abuse; and therapeutic drug monitoring. Increasingly sophisticated analytic methods are available to accomplish these tasks, but it is imperative that they be used judiciously. The numbers of compounds for which true emergency laboratory results are needed to guide therapy are still relatively few. For most potentially lethal intoxications the victim must be treated empirically before the laboratory results are known. A wide held misconception is that the laboratory can routinely detect any of the thousands of potential drugs or toxins that may be present in a sample. Because the financial and personnel resources required for such complete "screens" would be prohibitive, clinical laboratories must employ selective procedures suitable for the victim population in question. Therefore in most cases in clinical or hospital-based settings, tests are done for only a finite number of compounds, generally the more common drugs of abuse. Ideally, a diagnosis of poisoning would be made clinically, with the laboratory playing a confirmatory role. This short chapter is meant to discuss the basic structures which are said to be vital in clinical toxicology laboratory.

The Role of Clinical Toxicology Laboratory

Most poisoned victims can be treated successfully without any contribution from the laboratory other than routine clinical biochemistry and hematology. This is particularly true for those cases where there is no doubt about the poison involved and when the results of a quantitative analysis would not affect therapy. However, toxicological analyses can play a useful role;

If the diagnosis is in doubt,

The administration of antidotes or protective agents is contemplated, or The use of active elimination therapy is being considered Drug monitoring.

Basic Information Necessary for Toxicology Laboratory

Close communication between clinical and laboratory personnel is essential. At a minimum, the ordering requisition for a toxicology screen should contain the following information.

A. Suspected agent(s)

The content of toxicology screens varies among laboratories. Although a standard screen may not include the suspected agent, if alerted beforehand the laboratory may be able to modify procedures as needed in order to search for the suspected agents.

B. Suspected dose

Analytic sensitivities vary among laboratories, and some facilities may not be able to detect therapeutic concentrations of certain drugs in their routine screens. Knowledge of the approximate dose ingested is important because in certain cases the use of analytic methods designed for therapeutic monitoring, not screening may be necessary.

C. Time of ingestion and sampling

Knowledge of both ingestion and sampling time is necessary to determine the degree of drug absorption; with serial determinations, knowledge of sampling times is critical, as a single quantitative level may be misleading and must be correlated with the time of ingestion. Serial levels, timed appropriately with respect to the pharmacokinetics of the agent, document that the concentration has peaked, which helps guide further therapy.

D. Clinical presentation

Knowledge of the clinical presentation helps the laboratory select the most appropriate screening procedures. The screening procedure for a victim with a depressed level of consciousness is entirely different from conscious victim.

E. Location of the victim

Location of the victim to the clinical laboratory determines the type of the test that is going to be done (e. g depending on its simplicity).

Steps in Undertaking an Analytical Toxicological Investigation

The analysis dealings with a case of poisoning are usually divided into pre-analytical, analytical and post-analytical phases

Pre-analytical phase

Obtain details of current admission, including any circumstantial evidence of poisoning and results of biochemical and hematological investigations

Obtain victim's medical history, if available, ensure access to the appropriate sample(s), and decide the priorities for the analysis.

Analytical phase

Perform the agreed analyses.

Post-analytical phase

Interpret the results and discuss them with the clinician looking after the victim.

Perform additional analyses, if indicated, on the original samples or on further samples from the victim.

Laboratory Specimens

Before starting an analysis it is important to obtain as much information about the victim as possible (medical, social and occupational history, treatment given, and the results of laboratory or other investigations). It is also important to be aware of the time that elapsed between ingestion or exposure and the collection of specimens, since this may influence the interpretation of results.

No single specimen type is universally appropriate for identification of toxic agents. The selection of specimen type is based on both the toxicokinetics of the suspected agent and laboratory methodology. In general, quantitative tests are performed on serum or whole blood, and qualitative tests are performed on urine and gastric contents. When in doubt, obtain as many specimen types as possible and forward to the laboratory, where the most appropriate specimens can be selected. For the broadest possible screening (which, again, is rarely needed, especially in emergency toxicology), minimally, blood and urine should be sent (detailed practical aspects of analytical toxicology is discussed in the next chapters).

A. Specimen collection

Urine

Urine is useful for screening tests as it is often available in large volumes and usually contains higher concentrations of drugs or other poisons than blood. The presence of metabolites may sometimes assist identification. A 50-ml specimen from an adult, collected in a sealed, sterile, plastic container, is sufficient for most purposes; no preservative should be added. Urine can be collected in acid washed, metal free container for quantification of heavy metals. The sample should be obtained as soon as possible, ideally before any drug therapy is initiated. Conversely, little poison may remain in specimens taken many hours or days later, even though the victim may be very ill, as in the case acute paracetamol poisoning.

Stomach contents

Stomach contents may include vomit, gastric aspirate and stomach washings - it is important to obtain the first sample of washings, since later samples may be very dilute. A volume of at least 20 ml is collected in plastic container to carry out a wide range of tests; no preservative should be added. It is the best sample on which to perform certain tests. If obtained soon after ingestion, large amounts of poison may be present while metabolites, which may complicate some tests, are usually absent. An immediate clue to certain compounds may be given by the smell; it may be possible to identify tablets or capsules simply by inspection.

Scene residues (non-biological)

It is important that all bottles or other containers and other suspect materials found with or near the victim (scene residues) are retained for analysis if necessary since they may be related to the poisoning episode.

A few milligrams of scene residues are usually sufficient for the tests described here. Dissolve solid material in a few milliliters of water or other appropriate solvent. Use as small amount as possible in each test, in order to conserve sufficient amount for possible further tests.

Blood

Blood (plasma or serum) is normally reserved for quantitative assays but for some poisons, such as carbon monoxide, whole blood has to be used for qualitative tests. Specimen should be collected in a sealed heparinized tube on admission. In addition, 2-ml sample should be collected in a fluoride/oxalate tube.

The use of disinfectant swabs containing alcohols (ethanol, propan-2-ol) should be avoided. In general, there are no significant differences in the concentrations of poisons between plasma and serum.

B. Specimen transport and storage

Specimens sent for analysis must be clearly labeled with the victim's full name, the date and time of collection, and the nature of the specimen. This is especially important if large numbers of victims have been involved in a particular incident, or a number of specimens have been obtained from one victim. The date and time of receipt of all specimens by the laboratory should be recorded and a unique identifying number assigned to each specimen. Containers of volatile materials, such as organic solvents, should be packaged separately from biological specimens to avoid the possibility of cross-contamination. All biological specimens should be stored at 4°C prior to analysis. Ideally any specimen remaining after the analysis should be kept at 4°C for 3-4 weeks in case further analyses are required. In view of the medico-legal implications of some poison cases (for example, if it is not clear how the poison was administered or if the victim dies) then any specimen remaining should be kept (preferably at -20°C) until investigation of the incident has been concluded.

C. Specimen examination

Urine

High concentrations of some drugs or metabolites can impart characteristic colors to urine. Treatment given for poisoning may color urine (E.g. Deferoxamine in iron poisoning color urine red or methylene blue given in treatment of nitrate poisoning may color urine blue). Strong-smelling poisons such as methylsalicylate can sometimes recognized in urine since they are excreted in part unchanged. Turbidity may be due to underlying pathology (blood, microorganisms, casts, epithelial cells), or carbonates, phosphates or urates (in amorphous or microcrystalline forms). Such findings should not be ignored, even though they may not be related to the poisoning.

Stomach contents and scene residues

Some characteristic smells can be associated with particular poisons (e. g alcohol). Very low or very high pH may indicate ingestion of acid or alkali, while a green/blue color suggests the presence of iron or copper salts. Microscopic examination using a polarizing microscope may reveal the presence of tablet or capsule debris. Undegraded tablets or capsules and any plant remains or specimens of plants thought to have been ingested should be examined separately.

Apparatus, Reference Compounds & Reagents

A. Apparatus

Analytical toxicology services can be provided in clinical biochemistry laboratories that serve a local hospital or accident and emergency unit. In addition to basic laboratory equipment, some specialized apparatus, such as that for thin-layer chromatography, ultraviolet and visible spectrophotometry and microdiffusion, is needed. A continuous mains electricity supply is not essential. No reference has been made to the use of more complex techniques, such as gas-liquid and high-performance liquid chromatography, atomic absorption spectrophotometry or immunoassays, even if simple methods are not available for particular compounds. Although such techniques are more selective and sensitive than many simple methods, there are a number of factors, in addition to operator expertise, that have to be considered before they can be used in individual laboratories.

The standards of quality (purity or cleanliness) of laboratory reagents and glassware and of consumable items such as solvents and gases needs to be considerably higher than for the tests described in this manual if reliable results are to be obtained. Additional complications, which may not be apparent when instrument purchase is contemplated, include the need to ensure a regular supply of essential consumables (gas chromatographic septa, injection syringes, chromatography columns, solvent filters, chart or integrator paper, recorder ink or fibre-tip pens) and spare or additional parts (detector lamps, injection loops, column packing materials). The instruments must be properly maintained.

Some drug-testing techniques are now available in kit form. For example, there are standardized thin-layer chromatography (TLC) drug screening systems. Similarly, immunoassay kits are relatively simple to use, although problems can arise in practice, especially in the interpretation of results. Moreover, they are aimed primarily at the therapeutic drug monitoring and drug abuse testing markets and, as such, have limited direct application in clinical toxicology.

B. Reference compounds and reagents

A supply of relatively pure compounds for use as reference standards is essential if reliable results are to be obtained.

However, expensive reference compounds of a very high degree of purity, such as those marketed for use as pharmaceutical quality control standards, are not normally needed. Some drugs, such as barbiturates, caffeine and salicylic acid, and many inorganic and organic chemicals and solvents are available as laboratory reagents with an adequate degree of purity through normal laboratory chemical suppliers. Such a reference collection is a valuable resource, and it should be stored under conditions that ensure safety, security and stability.

Although the apparatus required to perform the tests described in this manual is relatively simple, several unusual laboratory reagents are needed in order to be able to perform all the tests described. At last, it is beyond the scope of the lecture note to cover all the reagents.

General Laboratory Tests in Clinical Toxicology

Many clinical laboratory tests can be helpful in the diagnosis of acute poisoning and in assessing prognosis. More specialized tests may be appropriate depending on the clinical condition of the victim, the circumstantial evidence of poisoning and the past medical history.

A. Biochemical tests

Blood glucose

Determination of blood glucose is essential to know those toxic substances that affect blood glucose bio-transformation. A toxicant that causes hypoglycemia includes insulin, iron, acetyl salicylic acid & so on.

Hyperglycemia is a less common complication of poisoning than hypoglycemia, but has been reported after over dosage with acetylsalicylic acid, salbutamol and theophylline.

Electrolytes, blood gases and pH

Toxic substances or their metabolites, which inhibit key steps in intermediary bio-transformation, are likely to cause metabolic acidosis owing to the accumulation of organic acids, notably lactate.

Measurement of the serum or plasma anion gap can be helpful. The anion gap is usually calculated as the difference between the sum of sodium & potassium concentration and the sum of the chloride and bicarbonate concentrations $((Na^+ + k^+) + (Cl^- + HCO3))$.

It is normally about 10mmol/l.

If arterial blood gas measurement is performed, direct measurement of oxygen saturation with a CO-oximeter allows detection of methemoglobin, resulting from intoxication with various oxidizing drugs or Carbon monoxide-hemoglobin

Plasma enzymes

The plasma activities of liver enzymes, such as aspartate aminotransferase, alanine aminotransferase may increase rapidly after absorption of toxic doses of substances that can cause liver necrosis, notably paracetamol, carbon tetrachloride, and copper salts.

Cholinesterase activity

Plasma cholinesterase is a useful indicator of exposure to organophosphorus compounds or carbamates, and a normal plasma cholinesterase activity effectively excludes acute poisoning by these compounds.

The diagnosis can sometimes be assisted by detection of a poison or metabolite in a body fluid, but the simplest method available is relatively insensitive.

Measurement of serum osmolality

The normal osmolality of plasma (280-295mOsm/Kg) is largely accounted by sodium, urea &glucose. However, large increases in plasma osmolality may follow the absorption of osmotically active poisons (especially methanol, ethanol, or propan-2-ol) in relatively large amounts. Together with the standard chemistry panel, serum osmolality allows identification of an osmolal gap, which may indicate intoxication with ethanol or other alcohols.

Osmolal gap can be calculated:

Osmolsl gap (Osmolarity) = 2(Na+) + Glucose ÷18 + BUN ÷ 2.8

B. Hematological tests

Hematocrit (Erythrocyte volume fraction)

Acute or acute-on-chronic over dosage with iron salts, acetylsalicylic acid, indomethacin, and other non-steroidal anti-inflammatory drugs may cause gastrointestinal bleeding leading to anemia.

Anaemia may also result from chronic exposure to toxins that interfere with haem synthesis, such as lead.

Leukocyte count

Increases in the leukocyte (white blood cell) count often occur in acute poisoning, for example, in response to an acute metabolic acidosis, resulting from ingestion of ethylene glycol or methanol, or secondary to hypostatic pneumonia following prolonged coma.

Blood clotting

The prothrombin time and other measures of blood clotting are likely to be abnormal in acute poisoning with rodenticides such as Coumarin anticoagulants.

Carboxyhemoglobin

Measurement of blood carboxyhemoglobin can be used to assess the severity of acute carbon monoxide poisoning.

However, carboxyhemoglobin is dissociated rapidly once the victim is removed from the contaminated atmosphere, especially if oxygen is administered, and the sample should therefore be obtained as soon as possible after admission. Even then, blood carboxyhemoglobin concentrations tend to correlate poorly with clinical features of toxicity.

17

Practical Aspects of Analytical Toxicology

Methods for particular toxicologic tests or panels are a well established part of routine laboratory tests, and information about them is available on request. In order to interpret toxicology results properly, the laboratory technician should have a rudimentary familiarity with the analytic methods employed. Several methods exist, varying in sensitivity, specificity, assay time, and cost. The choice depends on the size and budget of the institution, the types of victims served the proximity to more elaborate toxicology facilities, and other factors. This chapter focuses on the practical aspects of analytical toxicology.

Selection of Test Methods

Selection of test methods can be generally classified as either screening or confirmatory.

I. Screening methods

Screening is the testing or examining of a poisoned person for a chemical agent causing toxicity. Screening methods are generally qualitative, relatively simple and inexpensive, and designed to maximize sensitivity (possibly with some sacrifice of specificity). No standard toxicology screening tests exists. Currently the most widely used screening tests are based on immunoassay methods. Screening methods, give the emphasis on maximizing sensitivity, may produce significant numbers of false-positive results.

A "negative" screen can rule out only the finite number of compounds tested for at concentrations above the threshold of detection for the particular method used. Because of the inherent limitations of screening tests, definitive results must be based on a second method, a confirmatory procedure. It is important to note that inclusion of chemicals in a screening panel is generally governed by methodological as well as clinical considerations.

Reporting & interpretation of toxicology screening results Toxicology screen results are usually reported with a list of the chemicals tested for and a comment regarding detection or presence of the chemicals.

1. *Positive screens:* The notation "toxin detected" is entered next to the particular chemicals found.
2. *Negative screens:* The notation "toxin tested for not detected" or similar comment is made. Negative toxicology screen results in the face of strong clinical suspicions to the contrary may occur due to a number of reasons.

a. Toxins clinically suspected and in fact present in a victim are not tested for. Thus a seemingly negative toxicology screen result is misleading. If laboratory personnel are notified of the suspected agents, they can generally either modify the existing screen or suggest alternative strategies.

b. The toxicology screen is performed on a specimen collected at a time outside the detection period for a particular toxin. Most of the common drugs of abuse are detectable in urine for 48-72 hours after ingestion, e.g., opiates

c. The toxins may be present in concentrations below the limits of detectability for the method used.

In general, when faced with an unresponsive victim and an incomplete clinical history, minimum testing should include quantification of ethanol, acetaminophen, salicylate, and barbiturates.

II. Confirmatory methods

Confirmatory methods are designed to have near-perfect specificity and tend to be technically much more complex and demanding. Confirmatory methods are of relatively little importance in the context of emergency toxicology. Their principal use is in legal situations, where it must be established beyond a reasonable doubt that a particular drug was present. In these cases, integrity of specimen handling (chain of custody) becomes as important as the analytic procedure itself in order to rule out the possibility of specimen tampering or substitution.

Common Analytical Toxicology Laboratory Techniques

I. Spot tests

Spot tests are rapid, easily performed, non-instrumental qualitative procedures. They are the most rudimentary toxicology tests, & generally performed on urine specimens. In the test procedure, the sample (that is suspected for having a particular toxic chemical) will react with a chemical or chemicals set as a solution, or coated on a strip & the result of the reaction expressed by a color formation detected visually or colorometrically.

Spot tests are available for a number of compounds, including salicylate, acetaminophen, carbonmonoxide, halogenated hydrocarbons, and heavy metals. The tests are rapid and convenient; however sensitivity and specificity are generally poor and accurate quantification is virtually impossible. Because of improvements in other technologies, spot tests are now largely replaced by rapid immuno- assays that may perform at the point-of-care or in the central laboratories.

II. Ultraviolet & visible spectrophotometry

Many toxins have characteristic absorption spectra, but they must be extracted from body fluids in order to measure these spectra. A number of the quantitative methods employ ultraviolet (UV) (200-400 nm) or visible (400-800 nm) spectrophotometry. The major problem encountered with this technique is interference, and some form of sample purification, such as solvent extraction or microdiffusion, is usually employed. For some drugs (e.g.,barbiturates, benzodiazepines and theophylline) the method offers reasonable sensitivity and specificity, but it is much less powerful and versatile than chromatographic method.

III. Immunoassays

Immunoassays are diagnostic techniques used for the detection of antigen and antibody. Depending on the immunoassay techniques that are employed for the specific test, either antigen or antibody may be detected from the samples based on their reaction with their specific antibody or antigen respectively.

Many types of immunoassay configuration can be devised. Those not involving radioactivity or separation steps (homogeneous immunoassays) can be automated on routine clinical chemistry instruments, making them convenient for laboratories of all sizes. Immunoassay techniques used to screening specimens for chemicals include: Enzyme-Multiplied immunoassay (EMIA), Florescence polarization Immunoassay (FPIA), Cloned enzyme donor Immunoassay (CEDIA), and Radio Immunoassay (RIA). Immunoassays can be made highly sensitive and quite specific, but their specificity is never absolute. Molecules with a similar structure generally cross-react to some degree, and occasionally substances interfere with the assay in some other fashion.

Immunoassays also have the drawback that each analyte must be individually assayed using an available antibody reagent. Nevertheless, some of the more modern, discrete analyzers can readily perform multiple homogenous immunoassays with minimal operator intervention, so a panel of commonly abused drugs (e.g., barbiturates, cocaine, opiates, cannabinoids, amphetamines, benzodiazepines) can be readily tested.

Immunoassay techniques have also been modified for on-site testing in the emergency department and other out victim settings. These tests are known as drug dipsticks; and they utilize paper strips impregnated with drug-specific antibody. The specimen is applied to the paper, and reagents produce a color development.

IV. Chromatography

Chromatography is a powerful technique for separating substances based on slight differences in chemical properties. In this method, components to be separated are distributed between two phases; as stationary and mobile phases.

Chromatographic procedure involve a sample to be introduced in a flowing stream of gas or liquid (mobile phase) that pass through a bed, layer, or column containing a stationary phase (made from solid, or gel or a liquid). As the mobile phase carries the sample pass the stationary phase, the solutes with lesser affinity remain in the mobile phase & travel faster & separate from those that have great affinity for it. Different chemicals have different characteristic mobility in a particular chromatographic system, allowing fairly confident identification.

In contrast to immunoassays, small chemical changes (e.g., addition or removal of a methyl group), commonly cause substantial changes in chromatographic mobility. Thus the parent drug can usually be distinguished from its metabolites.

Types of chromatographic techniques

a. Thin-layer chromatography (TLC)

TLC has been widely used for urine toxicology. It does not require special equipment, is suitable for analysis of large batches of samples, is available in commercial kit form, and allows use of various color reagents in addition to chromatographic mobilities to aid in chemical identification. TLC, however, is too slow and cumbersome to be readily applied to emergency toxicology, and it is generally not quantitative. Its sensitivity is relatively poor.

b. Gas chromatography (GC) and high-performance liquid chromatography (HPLC)

are powerful techniques requiring dedicated equipment and skilled operators, but they can be adapted to a wide range of screening or quantitative assays.

Gas chromatography

GC is the technique of choice for volatile agents (ethanol, methanol, isopropanol, ethylene glycol). Use of open tubes (capillaries) allows rapid, high-resolution separations. Many detection methods can be applied, some with high sensitivity; and definitive drug identification is possible by coupling the GC with mass spectrometry.

HPLC

HPLC has been developed more recently than GC, is a more natural technique for the analysis of nonvolatile compounds. Modern columns perform highly efficient separations, although resolution is not as good as that of GC. Detection is usually by ultraviolet spectrophotometry, which in its most sophisticated form permits spectral scanning of each eluting peak to aid in identification.

V. Mass spectrometry and other specialized techniques

Mass spectrometry is an analytical instrument that first ionizes a target molecule and then separates and measures the mass of a molecule or its fragment. The analysis is qualitative, quantitative & extremely useful for determining the elemental composition & structure of both inorganic & organic compounds.

When mass spectroscopy (MS) is coupled to gas chromatography (GC-MS), nearly full proof chemical identification is possible because substances are identified from both their retention time measured by GC and their characteristic fragmentation pattern on MS. Using computer-based libraries of fragmentation patterns, GC-MS can be used to screen a wide variety of drugs simultaneously. Despite the availability of affordable bench-top instruments, however, GC-MS remains too sophisticated for routine application in clinical toxicology, although it has tremendous importance as the essential confirmatory technique in forensic toxicology.

VI. Nuclear magnetic resonance (NMR)

NMR is another technique that can perform both definitive substance identification and screening of body fluid, although at a much lower sensitivity than GC-MS. The technique, however, is even more expensive than GC-MS.

VII. Atomic absorption, plasma emission, neutron activation, and x-ray fluorescence, Toxic metals, for which most of the previously discussed methods do not apply, can be analyzed by sophisticated spectroscopic techniques, including atomic absorption, plasma emission, neutron activation, and x-ray fluorescence.

18

Toxicants of Public Health Hazard

The rapid industrialization and successful green revolution have introduced a large variety of chemicals into our environment. The species and varieties of environmental chemicals are as many as we can visualize. We may however, characterize them as: industrial chemicals which include organic and inorganic substances, metals, gases, fumes, solvents, and intermediates; agrochemicals, a major input of farming industry, comprising a variety of pesticides, fertilizers and growth promoters; pharmaceuticals, in innumerable number; and food additives, plastics, cosmetics etc. These have caused a great danger and put human and environment at a high risk. This chapter is meant for discussion of some of the important toxicants of public health hazard.

Industrial Toxicants

Industrial chemicals causing diseases have existed ever since man began manufacturing on a large scale & during the industrial revolution occupational diseases became common. Many of the chemicals used in industry are chemically reactive molecules & are likely to interact with biological systems & cause damage in some cases at the site of exposure. Exposure is most commonly via skin & lungs. There are now many thousands of chemical substances used in industry ranging from metals & inorganic compounds which risk people who work with it.

A. Heavy metal poisoning

Some metals such as iron are essential for life, while others such as lead are present in all organisms but serve no useful biologic purpose. Some of the oldest diseases of humans can be traced to heavy metal poisoning associated with metal mining, refining and use. Heavy metals are found every where: including in food, air, water, etc.

Lead Poisoning

Lead poisoning is one of the oldest occupational and environmental diseases in the world. Despite its recognized hazards, lead continues to have widespread commercial application (like ingested lead paints, pica, and lead pipes etc...). Environmental lead exposure, ubiquitous by virtue of the anthropogenic distribution of lead to air, water and food, has declined considerably due to diminished use of lead in gasoline and other applications. Lead serves no useful purpose in the human body. Lead is slowly but consistently absorbed via the respiratory and gastrointestinal tracts. Inorganic lead is poorly absorbed through the skin Absorption via the GIT varies with the nature of the lead compound, but in general, adults absorb about 10% of the ingested amount while young children absorb closer to 50%. The daily lead consumption is about 300μg. It is unsafe if consumed at a concentration greater than 0.5 mg/day for 3 months or more. Once absorbed from the respiratory or GIT, lead is bound to erythrocytes and widely distributed initially to soft tissues, then to the subperiosteal surface of bone and bone matrix. It has a half- life of 2-3weeks in blood and 15 years in bone. More than 90% of the lead that is eliminated appears in the urine.

Lead exerts multi systemic toxic effects through at least three mechanisms by; Inhibiting enzyme activity (e. g Interference with enzymes responsible for hemesynthesis) (See the fig below).

Interfering with the action of essential cations, particularly calcium, iron, and zinc.

Altering the structure of cell membranes and receptors (e. g attachment of lead to RBC membranes'! increased fragility and decreased survival time due to interference of sodium-potassium pump).

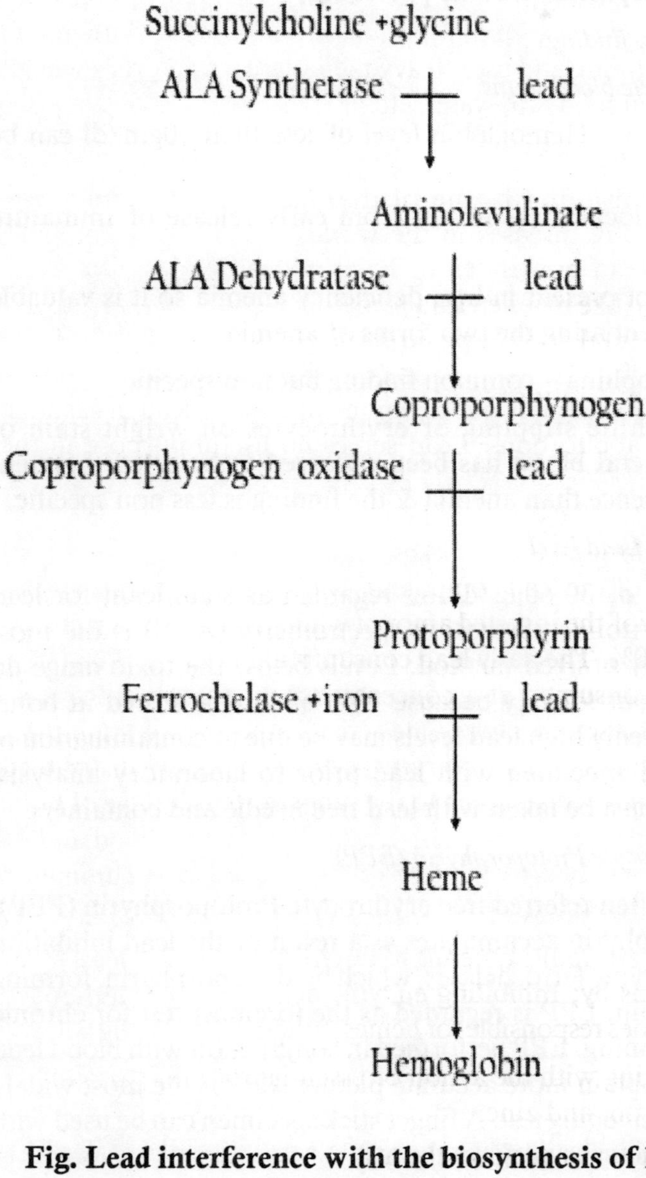

Fig. Lead interference with the biosynthesis of heme

The sign and symptoms of lead poisoning may include anorexia, apathy, behavioral changes, persistent vomiting, convulsions (acute poisoning) & ataxia, wrist & ankle drop, chronic nephritis (chronic poisoning)

Laboratory findings

A. Complete blood count

- Anemia – Hemoglobin level of less than 10gm/dl can be seen
- Reticulocytosis – results from early release of immature RBCs.

It is not present in iron deficiency anemia so it is valuable for differentiating the two forms of anemia.

- Eosinophilia – common finding but non specific
- Basophilic stippling of erythrocytes on wright stain of peripheral blood has been observed to be a less frequent occurrence than anemia & the finding is less non specific.

B. Serum Lead level

Levels of 30-60µg/dl are regarded as significant for lead toxicity. Atomic absorption spectrometry (AAS) is the most commonly utilized method. Levels below the toxic range do not rule out toxicity because 90% of lead is stored in bone. Unexpectedly high lead levels may be due to contamination of the blood specimen with lead prior to laboratory analysis. Sample must be taken with lead free needle and containers.

c. Erythrocyte Protoporphyrin (EPP)

EPP often referred free erythrocyte Protoporphyrin (FEP). Protoporphyrin accumulates as a result of the lead inhibition of the enzyme ferrochelases, which binds to porphyrin, forming hemoglobin. EPP is regarded as the foremost test for chronic lead poisoning. EPP performed in conjunction with blood lead levels to obtain more accurate picture. EPP is the most widely utilized screening test. A finger stick specimen can be used with a fluorometer to perform the test.

D. Delta-aminolevulinate dehydratase activity (ALA-D)

Lead decreases the activity of ALA-D, which is present in the erythrocytes. It is more sensitive than Protoporphyrin levels.

E. Urinary ALA and coproporphyrin III

Urinary levels of ALA are increased owing to lead inhibiting the enzyme ALA-D. Lead inhibition of the enzyme coproporphyrinogen oxidase has been proposed as a cause for increased coproporphyrin.

F. Calcium disodium versenate (CaNa2-EDTA) provocation test

CaNa2-EDTA administered to evaluate the chelatable lead store.

Specific laboratory tests

Qualitative test

Specimen

Stomach contents and scene residues

Reagents (see annex I)

1. Sodium tartrate buffer, pH 2.8.
2. Aqueous sodium rhodizonate solution (10 g/l).

Procedure

1. Add 0.1 ml of sodium tartrate buffer to 0.1 ml of test solution and vortex-mix for 5 seconds.
2. Spot 50 µl of acidified solution on to phase-separating filter-paper and add 50 µl of sodium rhodizonate solution.

Results

Lead salts give a purple colour in this test. However, the test is not specific: barium salts give a brown colour and a number of other metals also give coloured complexes.

Sensitivity

Lead, 2 mg/1

Quantitative tests

Principle

Whole blood that represents calibrators, controls, or victim specimens is mixed with ammonium phosphate and Triton X-100 to prepare it for graphite furnace atomic absorption analysis. The final step of analysis causes vaporization of lead, which absorbs energy at the 283.2nm light emitted from a hollow cathode lamp. Absorbance of energy at this wavelength is specific for lead and proportional to its concentration. Exposure of the specimen to high chloride concentration is to be avoided, because the chloride salt of lead is volatile at the charring temperatures used in atomic absorption analysis (Annex II).

Reagents (see Annexure I)

1. Ultra pure concentrated nitric acid.
2. Diluent (matrix modifier)
3. Calibrators
4. Controls. Commercial whole blood control.

Procedure

1. The first two specimens analyzed represent blanks. They consist of 0.25 mL of triple-distilled water and 1.0 mL of diluent.
2. Calibrating solutions are made by mixing 1.0 mL of the diluent with 0.25 mL of each calibrator.
3. The control pool and victim specimens are prepared for analysis by mixing 0.25 mL of each sample with 1.0 mL of diluent.
4. Add 10 µL of matrix modifier to 10µL of each sample and inject into the L'vov platform.
5. Record the absorbance peak area generated by each specimen. Repeat the analysis at an appropriate dilution for any specimen with an absorbance greater than that of the high concentration calibrator.

Calculation

1. Subtract the blank absorbance peak area from each specimen absorbance peak area.

2. Perform a best-fit regression analysis of the calibrator concentrations versus the respective absorbance peak area to define the calibration curve.

Compare the absorbance peak area derived from each specimen against the calibration curve to determine the concentration of lead. If the results among duplicates vary by more than 10%, sample contamination during processing is likely to have occurred.

Management

Chelating agents (Antidotes) E.g. dimercaprol, CaNa2-EDTA

Symptomatic management

Hydrocarbon Poisoning

Hydrocarbon comprises a broad group of organic compounds that contain hydrogen & carbon atoms only. Most, but not all, are derived from petroleum distillation. Hydrocarbons are found alone or incombination with others in a wide variety of commercial products ubiquitous around the home or work place. Lighter fluid, paint thinners, &removers, some furniture polishes, cleaning agents, solvents, various automotive products and ordinary fuels are common examples. These agents were the most frequently involved substances in human exposures, accounting for almost 5% of all poisoning .The overall mortality rate for accidental ingestion of these agents is difficult to estimate but may approach 0.5%. Modes of toxicity vary with age. Most cases involve accidental imbibing by young children. Abuse by inhalation is generally seen in male adolescents & young adults. The most common substances reported in toxic ingestions are gasoline, kerosene, mineral seal oil preparations, &lighter fluid. Most victims who are exposed to hydrocarbon develop pulmonary symptoms due to aspiration pneumonitis. It is clear that non-pulmonary manifestations like CNS toxicity, GI signs, and cutaneous signs are distinctly uncommon.

Lab Studies

- Routine laboratory tests are of little value for purposes of screening victims for admission.

- Arterial blood gas analysis (ABGs) must be measured in all victims with respiratory symptoms. Varying degrees of hypoxia without hypercarbia are the most common finding.
- Occasionally a metabolic acidosis is seen.
- The CBC may show leukocytosis
- Blood hydrocarbon levels are not readily available &have little diagnostic, prognostic, or therapeutic value. Qualitative testing is occasionally needed for forensic purposes.

Specific tests

Qualitative test

Reagents

1. Sodium hydroxide solution(20%,w/v, aqueous)
2. Pyridine
3. Positive control (dissolve 500mg chloral hydrate in 100ml of ethanol.)

Procedure

1. Take 1ml of the urine sample in a test tube
2. Add 1ml of 20% NaOH & 1ml of pyridine
3. Heat in a boiling water bath for 1 minute
4. A pink red color in the pyridine layer indicates the presence of hydrocarbon.

Pesticides

Pesticides are any substance or mixture of substances intended for preventing, destroying, repelling or mitigating any pest. Pesticide can be divided into several groups, such as insecticides, rodenticides, fungicides & herbicides. This part will give attention to the most frequent pesticide poisoning.

1. Insecticides

Organophosphates & carbamates are the most frequently used insecticides worldwide. These compounds cause 80% of the reported toxic exposure to insecticides.

Organophosphurus insecticides

These agents are utilized to combat a large variety of pests. Some of these agents are used in human and veterinary medicine as local or systemic antiparasitics or in circumstances in which prolonged inhibition of cholinesterase is indicated. The compounds are absorbed by the skin as well as by the respiratory and GITs. Biotransformation is rapid. In mammals as well as insects, the major effect of these agents is inhibition of acetyl cholinesterase. The signs and symptoms that characterize acute intoxication are due to inhibition of this enzyme resulting in accumulation of acetylcholine (diarrhea, urination, miosis, bradycardia, lacrimations &salivation).

Laboratory analysis

1. Serum electrolytes (e.g. Hypokalemia, hyperglycemia), Blood urea nitrogen, creatinine, CBC (e.g. leukocytosis secondary to increased catecholamine release from the adrenal medulla), urinalysis (e.g. Proteinuria and glycosuria), amylase level (elevated due to pancreatic injury), plasma and RBC cholinesterase levels
2. Toxic – specific findings

- Plasma and RBC cholinesterase levels are depressed
- Depression of RBC cholinesterase level is more specific for organophosphate poisoning and parallels the activity of neurosynaptic cholinesterase
- Plasma cholinesterase levels are a less specific but more

sensitive measure of toxicity

Specific tests Qualitative test Specimen

Stomach contents, scene residues.

Reagents

1. Sodium bicarbonate (solid)
2. Cyclohexane:acetone:chloroform (70:25:5)
3. Acetone:tetraethylenepentamine (9:1)
4. 4-(p- Nitrobenzyl) pyridine (20 g/1) in acetone: tetraethylenepentamine (9:1).

5. Silica gel thin-layer chromatography plate (5 × 20 cm, 20 μm average particle size).

Procedure

1. Carefully adjust the pH of 10 ml of sample to about 7 by adding solid sodium bicarbonate.
2. Extract 10 ml of sample with 5 ml of methyl tertiary-butyl ether for 5 minutes using a rotary mixer.
3. Allow to stand for 5 minutes, take off the upper, ether layer and re-extract with a second 5-ml portion of methyl tertiary-butyl ether.
4. Combine the extracts, filter through phase-separating filter-paper into a clean tube and evaporate to dryness under a stream of compressed air or nitrogen.
5. Analyze the final solution in thin layer chromatography (see Annexure I-number 3)

Results

The compounds of interest give purple spots on a pale brown background.

Sensitivity

Organophosphorus pesticide, 5 mg/l

Confirmatory test

Confirmatory test for organophosphorus pesticide is cholinesterase activity test.

Specimen

Plasma or serum

Cholinesterase activity monograph

Qualitative test

Specimen

Plasma or serum

Reagents (see annex I-number 7)

1. Dithiobisnitrobenzoate reagent.
2. Aqueous acetylthiocholine iodide solution.
3. Aqueous pralidoxime chloride solution.
4. Plasma or serum from an unexposed individual (control plasma).

Procedure

1. Add 2.0 ml of dithiobisnitrobenzoate reagent and 1.0 ml of acetylthiocholine iodide solution to each of three 10-ml test-tubes.
2. Add 20 μl of control plasma to one tube and 20 μl of test plasma to a second.
3. Add 20 μl of pralidoxime solution and 20 μl of test plasma to the third tube.
4. Vortex-mix the contents of all three tubes and allow to stand at room temperature for 2 minutes.

Results

The presence of an acetylcholinesterase inhibitor is indicated if the yellow colour in the control tube is deeper than in the test tube. If the colour in the tube containing pralidoxime is similar to that in the control tube, this provides further confirmation that an inhibitor of acetylcholinesterase is present in the sample. Inhibitors of acetylcholinesterase, such as many carbamate pesticides, also give a positive result in this test.

Treatment

GI decontamination

Dermal decontamination

Symptomatic treatment

Toxin-specific like atopine, pralidoxime

Carbamate pesticides

Produce a milder form of toxicity, similar to that produced by organophosphate compounds. These compounds inactivate acetylcholinesterase leading to excessive accumulation of acetylcholine. The important differences distinguishing carbamates from organophosphate toxicity are

- Carbamate toxicity is typically short-lived in which spontaneous regeneration of enzymatic activity usually occur within 24 hours
- Carbamates produce little or no CNS toxicity because of their inability to penetrate the blood-brain-barrier & affect brain cholinesterase activity

Sign & symptoms may be more rapid &usually abate within 24 hrs regardless of therapy

Laboratory findings

RBC &plasma cholinesterase measurement not useful due to minimal &transient effects on these levels

Qualitative test

Specimen

Stomach contents, scene residues.

Reagents

1. Aqueous hydrochloric acid (2 mol/l)
2. Furfuraldehyde solution (100 ml/l) in methanol, freshly prepared.
3. Concentrated hydrochloric acid (relative density 1.18).

Procedure

1. Acidify 1 ml of sample with 0.5 ml of dilute hydrochloric acid and extract with 4 ml of chloroform on a rotary mixer for 5 minutes.
2. Centrifuge for 5 minutes, discard the upper, aqueous layer and filter the chloroform extract through phase-separating filter-paper into a clean tube.
3. Evaporate the extract to dryness under a stream of compressed air or nitrogen at 40°C.
4. Dissolve the residue in 0.1 ml of methanol, apply a spot of the solution to filter-paper and allow drying.

5. Apply 0.1 ml of furfuraldehyde solution to the spot;
6. Allow drying and exposing the paper to concentrated hydrochloric acid fumes for 5 minutes in a fume cupboard.

Results

Carbamates give a black spot. Non-pesticide carbamates can interfere in this test.

Sensitivity

Carbamate, 100 mg/l

Treatment

GI decontamination

Atropine, & pralidoxime can be used as an antidote

2. Rodenticides

Rodenticides are used to control rodent population. Anticoagulant preparations, currently the most widely used rodenticides, are safer, although consequential human poisonings do occur. Most pediatric ingestions occur accidentally, whereas ingestions in adults tend to be deliberate. Coumarin derivatives (e.g., warfarin) are one of the members of this class. Mechanism of action is by inducing coagulopathic state by inhibiting activation of the vitamin K - dependent clotting factors II, VII, IX and X. Victims are usually asymptomatic unless presentation is delayed over a period of several days, as the anticoagulant effects take place victims may experience spontaneous bleeding. The main features of warfarin poisoning in less severe cases are excessive bruising, nose & gum bleeding, &blood in the urine faeces. Bleeding from several organs within the body, leading to shock & possibly death, occurs in the more severe cases. The onset of the signs of poisoning may not be evident until a few days after exposure.

Laboratory analysis

- General tests
- Check a baseline prothrombin time (PT), partial prothrombin time (PTT) and CBC.

- Toxin-specific tests
- Recommended monitoring factor VII-X complex levels are sensitive indicators of toxicity
- Warfarin may be detected by gas chromatography

Specific laboratory tests

Quantitative test

Specimen Urine, plasma Procedure

HPLC method is used for the fluorometric determination of warfarin & its metabolites. The detection scheme utilizes post column acid- base fluorescence enhancement techniques that provide high chromatographic specificity &sensitivity. Detection limit are in the low nanogram range. Other procedures, like UV spectrometry &revised- phase liquid chromatography, with a detection limit in blood serum of 20μg/1.

Cynide Toxicity

Cyanide is a cellular poison that can readily bind to many enzymes, having metallic component especially cytochrome oxid as eaterminalenzyme involved in aerobic bio-transformation. Inhibition results in anoxia. Cyanide has been also shown to bind to many other proteins. Cyanide sources can be certain plants (E.g. cassava), cyanide gas (e.g. cigarette smoke), medicines that liberate cyanide (E.g. Nitroprusside), exposure in fires etc...Oral absorption of cyanide is rapid and the toxic effects can present within minutes. It is widely distribution in the body & about 80% eliminated through the kidney in a form of thiocyanate. Organs such as the brain and heart are affected particularly as they require ATP and have limited capacity to cope with a deficit. The heart has only enough ATP to last 3 minutes , hence, cyanide may cause death as a result of heart or respiratory failure. The sign and symptoms of cyanide poisoning include headache, hypoxic convulsion, and respiratory distress, cyanide odor.

Laboratory analysis

i. General tests

1. Chemistry Tests

- Because of the blockade of aerobic bio-transformation, cyanide produces an anion gap metabolic acidosis secondary to the production of lactic acid
- Glucose catabolism is also altered, and the blood glucose level may be elevated

2. Blood gas analysis

- PaO_2 and oxygen saturation are unaltered except in severe cases where respiratory failure occurs.
- pH and $PaCO_2$ are altered in different ways, depending on the severity of poisoning.

ii. Toxin – specific tests

1. A spot test is a quick bedside test that can qualitatively detect the presence of cyanide using gastric aspirate.
2. The specific cyanide level is the gold standard test and should be done even though the results may not be readily available. These levels are usually performed on whole blood but some laboratories use serum or plasma.

Specific laboratory tests

Qualitative test

Specimen

Stomach contents, scene residues.

N.B: specimens containing cyanides often evolve hydrogen cyanide if acidified.

Reagents

1. Aqueous sodium hydroxide solution (100 g/l).
2. Aqueous ferrous sulfate solution (100 g/l, freshly prepared in freshly boiled and cooled water).
3. Aqueous hydrochloric acid (100 ml/l).

Procedure

1. Dilute 1 ml of sample with 2 ml of sodium hydroxide solution.

2. Add 2 ml of ferrous sulfate solution.
3. Add sufficient hydrochloric acid to dissolve the ferrous hydroxide precipitate.

Result

A blue colour indicates the presence of cyanide.

Sensitivity

Cyanide, 10 mg/1

Quantitative assays

Specimen

Heparinized whole blood (0.1-1.0 ml),

N.B. The samples can be stored at 4°C for 1-2 days if the analysis is delayed for any reason. (Cyanide in blood is less stable if stored at room temperature or at -20°C.)

p-Nitrobenzaldehyde/ o-dinitrobenzene method

Reagents

1. Aqueous sodium hydroxide (0.5 mol/1).
2. Aqueous sulfuric acid (3.6 mol/1).
3. p-Nitrobenzaldehyde (0.05 mol/1) in 2-methoxyethanol.
4. o-Dinitrobenzene (0.05 mol/1) in 2-methoxyethanol.

Standard

Aqueous potassium cyanide (10 mg/1, i.e., cyanide ion concentration, 4 mg/1)

Method: microdiffusion method

1. Take three microdiffusion cells and add to each of the centre wells: (a) 0.5 ml of p-nitrobenzaldehyde solution; (b) 0.5 ml of o-dinitrobenzene solution; (c) 0.1 ml of sodium hydroxide solution
2. To the outer wells add 0.1 ml of:

- Purified water (cell 1);
- Potassium cyanide solution (cell 2);

- Test blood specimen (cell 3).
3. To each outer well add 0.5 ml of purified water and, on the opposite side of the outer well, 1.0 ml of dilute sulfuric acid.
4. Seal each well using silicone grease and carefully mix the components of the outer wells.
5. Incubate at room temperature for 20 minutes and then add 1 ml of aqueous methanol (1:1) to the centre wells.
6. Transfer the contents of the centre wells to 5.0-ml volumetric flasks and make up to volume with aqueous methanol (1:1).

Results

The red coloration obtained with cyanide-containing solutions is stable for about 15 minutes. Measure the absorbance of the solutions from cells 2 and 3 at 560 nm against the purified water blank (cell 1). Assess the cyanide ion concentration in the sample by comparison with the reading obtained from the standard.

Sensitivity

Cyanide, 0.5 mg/1

Treatments

Symptomatic management

Toxin specific measures

- Nitrite-thiosulfate, hydroxycobalamin

Toxicity of Household Products

The ingestion of household products by a child is the most common pediatric medical emergency. Most household products are of relatively low toxicity. The top household products ingested are cleaning agents, cosmetics & personal products & berries. The manifestations when they do occur usually consist of mild GI upset.

Bleach is perhaps the substance most commonly involved in poisoning cases. When bleach is ingested orally it causes burning to the throat, mouth & aesophagus. The tissue damage results in edema in the pharynx & larynx. In the stomach the presence of endogenous hydrochloric acid generates hypochlorous acid which is irritant & chlorine gas which may be inhaled causing toxic effects in the lungs.

Medical Toxicants

Drugs are biologically active molecules used in the treatment, prevention & diagnosis of disease. However, drugs have made & will continue to make a major contribution to human health, we must accept the risks attached to these benefit.

The basic mechanisms for the toxicities arising from drugs are;

- Direct& predictable toxic effects due to over doses
- Toxic effects occurring after repeated therapeutic doses
- Direct but unpredictable toxic effects occurring after single therapeutic doses due to idiosyncratic response (peculiar response of an individual to a drug).
- Toxic effects due to another drug or substance interfering with the disposition or pharmacological response.

So, we do have a short overview of some of the common medical toxicants.

A. Acetaminophen

Acetaminophen is analgesics for mild &moderate pain which is very safe provided only the normal therapeutic dose. Acetaminophen is one of the drugs most commonly involved in suicide and accidental poisoning. Initial symptoms after an overdose are mild and non specific, often resulting in delayed arrival for medical care or a missed diagnosis. Acute ingestion of more than 150-200mg/kg (children) or 7gm (adults) is considered potentially toxic. Paracetamol is metabolized mainly by conjugation & minor proportion metabolized by oxidation which produces toxic products which detoxified normally. However, overdoses change the metabolic scheme giving a rise in toxic metabolite which react with liver proteins & cause tissue damage (leading to hepatic toxicity). Initially, the victim is asymptomatic or has mild GI upset (nausea, vomiting) which is followed by evidence of liver injury.

Laboratory analysis

- Severity of poisoning is determined from serum acetaminophen level.
- Detection of bilirubin level and prothrombin time can tell prognosis
- Elevated aminotransferase levels can be seen
- Monitor blood glucose because in toxic cases hypoglycemia and hyperglycemia have been reported.
- The plasma creatinine rises more rapidly than BUN when renal failure is present. Liver failure may keep the BUN low.
- Serum amylase is determined because of reports of pancreatitis

Specific laboratory tests

Qualitative tests

Reagents (See Annexure I- number 8)

1. Saturated o-cresol.
2. Ammonium hydroxide, 4 mol/1
3. Concentrated hydrochloric acid.

Procedure

1. Mix 1 mL of specimen (victim or control urine, water blank) and 1 mL of concentrated hydrochloric acid. Heat at 1000C for 10 min.
2. Cool and add 100 μL of the above solution to 10 mL of o-cresol reagent and then 2 mL of ammonium hydroxide, 4 mol/1

Result

Acetaminophen is hydrolyzed to p-aminophenol, which reacts with o- cresol and ammonium hydroxide to form an indophenol blue chromogen.

Quantitative tests

Principle

Acetaminophen and 3-acetamidophenol, added as an internal standard, are extracted from serum and analyzed by reverse-phase HPLC with an octadecylsilane bonded-phase column. The peak height absorbance ratio for acetaminophen relative to the internal standard is determined at 254 nm.

Reagents (see Annexure I)

1. Acetaminophen stock reference solution
2. Calibrator. Acetaminophen 20 and 100 µg/mL.
3. 3-Acetamidophenol stock internal standard, 1000 mg/L.
4. 3-Acetaminophen working internal standard, 50 mg/ml.
5. Phosphate buffer.
6. Mobile phase: sodium acetate buffer/acetonitrile (92/8) by volume).

Procedure

1. Pipette 100 µL of each calibrator, control, and victim's serum into properly labeled 13 x 100-mm glass tubes.
2. Add 100 µL of working internal standard solution and 100 µl of phosphate buffer (0.225 mol/L, pH 7.4) mix.
3. Add 3mL of ethyl acetate. Mix in a Vortex mixer for 15 s.
4. Centrifuge all tubes at 1000 x g for 5 min.
5. Transfer the organic (top) layer to labeled 12 x 75-mm glass tubes and evaporate under a stream of dry air at 50 0C.
6. Reconstitute the contents of each tube with 100 µL of the mobile phase and inject 10 to 20 µL into the HPLC instrument.

Calculation

Determine the peak height (or peak area) ratios of acetaminophen relative to the internal standard. Calculate the concentration of acetaminophen in the unknown by comparing its peak height ratio versus acetaminophen concentration response for the calibrator.

Treatment

GI decontamination

Antidote (acetylcysteine)

B. Aspirin (salicylate)

Acetylsalicylic acid, commonly known as aspirin, is still one of the most widely used minor analgesics. Salicylate poisoning is a much less common cause of childhood poisoning deaths since the introduction of child-resistant container and the reduced use of baby aspirin. Salicylates, however still accounts for numerous suicidal and accidental poisonings. Salicylate Poisoning can also result from chronic over medication; this occurs most commonly in elderly victims using salicylates for chronic pain because of impaired biotransformation, excretion & others. Salicylic acid is then metabolized by conjugation. These conjugation steps are saturable so the half life of aspirin increases significantly with only small increase in the number of tablets. The first sign of salicylate toxicity is often hyperventilation and respiratory alkalosis due to medullary stimulation. Metabolic acidosis follows due to accumulation of intracellular lactate as well as excretion of bicarbonate by the kidney to compensate for respiratory alkalosis.

Laboratory tests

Urine should be tested for pH, the presence of ketone bodies and hemoglobin. A rapid qualitative test for the presence of salicylates may be done in urine. Serum measurements of salicylate are important after acute ingestions.

Specific laboratory tests Qualitative test Specimen Urine, stomach contents, scene residues.

Reagent (see Annexure I) Trinder's reagent

Procedure

Add 0.1 ml of Trinder's reagent to 2 ml of sample and mix for 5 seconds.

N.B. To test for acetylsalicylic acid or methyl salicylate in stomach contents or scene residues, and to test for salicylamide in urine, stomach contents or scene residues, first boil 1 ml of sample with 1 ml of aqueous hydrochloric acid (0.1 mol/l) for 10 minutes, & cool (filter if necessary), and then neutralize with 1 ml of aqueous sodium hydroxide (0.1 mol/l).

Results

A strong violet color indicates the presence of salicylates. Azide preservatives react strongly in this test, and weak false positives can be given by urine specimens containing high concentrations of ketone bodies.

This test is sensitive and will detect therapeutic dosage with salicylic acid, acetylsalicylic acid, 4-aminosalicylic acid, methyl salicylate and salicylamide.

Sensitivity

Salicylate, 10 mg/l

Quantitative assay

Specimen

Plasma or serum (1 ml)

Reagent

Trinder's reagent

Standards

Aqueous solutions containing salicylic acid at concentrations of 0, 200, 400 and 800 mg/l. Store at 4°C when not in use.

Procedure

1. Add 5 ml of Trinder's reagent to 1 ml of sample or standard.
2. Vortex-mix for 30 seconds and centrifuge for 5 minutes.
3. Measure the absorbance of the supernatant at 540 nm against plasma blank.

Results

Calculate the plasma salicylate concentration from the graph obtained on analysis of the salicylate standards. Some salicylate metabolites interfere, but plasma concentrations of these compounds are usually low. Oxalates, for example, from fluoride/ oxalate blood tubes, also interfere in this test.

Sensitivity

Salicylate, 50 mg/1

Treatment

GI decontamination

Facilitating diuresis

Symptomatic management

C. Barbiturates

Barbiturates belong to a class of sedative-hypnotic drugs with abuse potential & a recognized withdrawal syndrome. Toxic manifestations of barbiturates vary with the amount of ingestion, type of drug and time elapsed since ingestion. Lower doses of short acting barbiturates (E.g. pentobarbital) than the long-acting barbiturates (e.g. Phenobarbital) generally cause toxicity, but fatalities are more common with the latter. Mild intoxication resembles that of alcohol intoxication. Moderate intoxication is characterized by greater depression of mental status and severe intoxication causes coma.

Laboratory analysis

1. Plasma barbiturate (e.g. Phenobarbital) levels are helpful for making a diagnosis but of little value when predicting the severity of the over dose.
2. As with alcohol, chronic abusers of Phenobarbital may have elevated serum levels with little CNS depression.

Specific laboratory tests Quantitative assay Specimen

Whole blood, plasma or serum (5 ml)

Reagents (see Annexure I)

1. Borate buffer, pH 8.4.
2. Aqueous hydrochloric acid (2 mol/l)
3. Concentrated sulfuric acid (relative density 1.83).
4. Concentrated ammonium hydroxide (relative density 0.88).
5. Sodium sulfate/charcoal mixture.

Standards (see Annexure I)

Solutions containing barbital at concentrations of 5, 10, 25 and 50 mg/l in blank human plasma.

Procedure

1. Add 5 ml of sample, 2 ml of hydrochloric acid and 60 ml of diethyl ether to a 250-ml separating funnel.
2. Lubricate (with purified water) and insert the funnel and shake gently for 2 minutes.
3. After standing for 5 minutes, and then discard the lower aqueous phase, add the diethyl ether extract to 10 ml of borate buffer in a second separating funnel and mix for 1 minute.
4. Allow to stand for 5 minutes and again discard the lower, aqueous phase through the funnel tap.
5. Wash round the funnel with 5 ml of purified water; allow standing for 5 minutes and again discarding the lower, aqueous phase through the funnel tap.
6. Add about 4 g of sodium sulfate/charcoal mixture to the ether extract in the funnel, shake to disperse, and filter the extract through phase-separating filter-paper into a 150-ml conical flask.
7. Add a further 20 ml of diethyl ether to the separating funnel, shake and add to the extract in the flask through the filter funnel.
8. Evaporate the extract to dryness on a water-bath at 40°C under a stream of compressed air or nitrogen.
9. Add 5.0 ml of purified water to the dry extract in the flask, swirl gently and allow to stand for 5 minutes.
10. Filter the reconstituted extract through phase-separating filter-paper into a 12.5-cm test-tube.
11. Check the spectrophotometer zero at 240 nm using purified water in both sample and reference positions.

12. Add 4 ml of filtrate from the test-tube to a clean, dry cell, add 50 µl of concentrated ammonium hydroxide and mix using a plastic paddle. Check that the pH is about 10.
13. Quickly measure the absorbance at 240 nm against purified water blank. If necessary, accurately dilute a portion of the extract with purified water to bring the reading on to the scale, and record the magnitude of the dilution. If a scanning spectrophotometer is available, scan in the region 200-450 nm.
14. Repeat the reading or scan after 5 minutes.
15. Add 0.1 ml of concentrated sulfuric acid to the cell, mix using the plastic paddle, and check that the pH is about 2.
16. Repeat the reading (240 nm) or scan (200-450 nm).

Results

1. To perform a quantitative measurement, measure the difference between absorbance at pH 10 and at pH 2, construct a calibration graph by analysis of the standard barbiturate solutions, and calculate the barbiturate concentration in the sample.

   Alternatively, use the following formula: ((absorbance at pH 10) - (absorbance at pH 2) × Dilution factor (if any) × 25 = barbiturate (mg/1)

2. Sample volumes of less than 5 ml may be used, but there will be a corresponding loss of sensitivity unless "micro"-volume fused silica spectrophotometer cells are available.

Sensitivity

Barbiturate, 2 mg/1

Treatment

GI decontamination

Alkalinization of urine

Hemodialysis

Environmental Toxicants

Exposure of biological systems to chemicals may occur through environmental pollution of the atmosphere, water or soil. This results from industrial, agricultural & other human activities. Food born toxins derived from different microbes also can contribute in causing environmental intoxication. The atmosphere may be polluted by gases such as carbon monoxide & particulates.

a. Carbon monoxide poisoning

Carbon monoxide (CO) is a colorless, odorless gas that is ubiquitous because it is produced by the incomplete combustion of carbon compounds. The possibility of carbon monoxide poisoning is obvious for the victim of fire and smoke inhalation; but accidental and suicidal exposures are also common. The gas is readily absorbed across the alveolus and combines with hemoglobin with high affinity than oxygen. This displacement of oxygen from hemoglobin leads to a decrease in oxygen transport and causes tissue hypoxia. Elimination of carbon monoxide is predominantly through respiration; only about 1% is metabolized to carbon dioxide. Victims with mild to moderate CO poisoning often complain of headache, dizziness and nausea and vomiting. Severe poisoning may result in chest pain, dyspnea, syncope, seizures and coma.

Laboratory analysis

- Carboxyheamoglobin level – should be measured as early as possible to establish the diagnosis of carbon monoxide poisoning. Carboxyheamoglobin should be measured from blood sample using spectrophotometric methods. Although not as accurate, carboxyheamoglobin levels can be estimated from expired air using a breath analyzer for carbon monoxide.
- Arterial blood gas assays are poor indicators of carbon monoxide poisoning. The PaO2 is often normal, as it is a measure of oxygen dissolved in plasma, not a measure of oxygen bound to hemoglobin.

Specific laboratory tests

Qualitative test

Applicable to whole blood treated with heparin, edetic acid or fluoride/oxalate.

Reagent

Aqueous ammonium hydroxide (0.01 mol/l)

Procedure

Add 0.1 ml of blood to 2 ml of ammonium hydroxide solution and vortex-mix for 5 seconds.

Results

A pink tint in comparison with the colour obtained from a normal blood specimen suggests the presence of carboxyhaemoglobin. Cyanide may give a similar tint, but acute cyanide poisoning is generally much less common than carbon monoxide poisoning.

Sensitivity HbCO, 20% Quantitative assay

Specimen:whole blood treated with heparin, edetic acid or fluoride/oxalate.

Reagents

1. Aqueous ammonium hydroxide (1 ml/l).
2. Sodium dithionite (solid, stored in a desiccator).
3. A supply of pure carbon monoxide or carbon monoxide/nitrogen.
4. A supply of oxygen or compressed air.

Procedure

1. Add 0.2 ml of blood to 25 ml of ammonium hydroxide solution and mix.
2. Take three approximately equal portions: x, y and z. Keep portion x in a stoppered tube while the following procedures are performed:

a. Saturate portion y with carbon monoxide (to give 100% HbCO) by bubbling the gas through the solution for 5-10 minutes. Take care to minimize frothing.

b. Saturate portion z with oxygen by bubbling pure oxygen or compressed air through the solution for at least 10 minutes to remove all bound carbon monoxide (to give 0% HbCO). Again, take care to minimize frothing.

3. Add a small amount (about 20 mg) of sodium dithionite to each test solution (x, y and z) and also to 10 ml of ammonium hydroxide solution and mix well.

4. Measure the absorbance of solutions x, y and z against the dithionite-treated ammonium hydroxide solution at 540 nm and 579 nm.

Results

The percentage carboxyhemoglobin saturation (% HbCO can be calculated from the equation:

(A540/A579solution x) - (A540/A579solution z)%HbCO =

(A540/A579solution y) - (A540/A579solution z) × 100

Approximate normal values are:

(A540/A579 solution y) = 1.5, corresponding to 100% HbCO
(A540/A579 solution z) = 1.1, corresponding to 0% HbCO.

The hemoglobin content of blood varies from person to person, and thus the volume of diluents used may need to be altered. A dilution giving a maximum absorbance of about 1 absorbance unit at 540 nm is ideal.

N.B. - It is important to use sodium dithionite that has been freshly obtained or stored in a sealed container in desiccators, since this compound is inactivated by prolonged contact with moist air.

- This method is unreliable in the presence of other pigments such as methaemoglobin (indicated by a relatively high absorbance in the region 580-600 nm).
- Lipaemic blood specimens may give turbid suspensions, which also give unreliable results.

Sensitivity

HbCO, approximately 10%

Treatment

100% oxygen

b. Food – born toxins

A microbial toxin is a compound produced by a microorganism that acts to cause disease. Food poisoning syndromes result after ingestion of a wide variety of foods contaminated with pathogenic microorganisms or microbial toxins. The pathogenic organisms are Clostridium perferinges, Bacillus cereus, Escherichia coli, Closterdium botulinium and Vibrio cholerae. Preformed toxins are from Staphylococcus aureus, B.cereus and C.botulinum. The illnesses produced usually are not associated with fever or blood, pus, or mucus in the stools because it doesn't have tissue involvement. Most of them produce GI symptoms. Except for botulism and cholera, the clinical course of most of these food-borne toxin related illnesses is self-limiting.

Laboratory analysis

General tests

- CBC may reveal hemoconcentration (there will be increase in hematocrit level)
- Urinalysis shows a trace of protein
- Fecal leucocytes are absent in the presence of food- borne toxin induced illness
- Stool culture in general is not helpful for the diagnosis of microbial toxin intoxication. However, in a common source outbreak, examination of food, gastric contents, or stool may be useful.

Because the clinical course of poisoning with the following organisms is self-limited, preparing & identifying cultures is not cost-effective and rarely alters treatment plans. However, confirmatory tests may be warranted in the case of a mass outbreak of food poisoning. In such instances the following tests can be done.

1. S. aureus – Gram-stain of the suspected food and culture.

2. B. cereus - Bacteria count of 105 organisms per gram of food is suspicious for B. cereus because it is the normal fecal flora.
3. C. perferingens -anaerobic culture of the implicated foods can isolate C. perfringens.
4. E. coli - Stool culture identifies the presence of E. coli strains, but differentiation of the various strains of E.coli requires expensive animal testing, which is not cost effective.

Toxin – specific tests

- Cholera – dark field microscopic examination of fresh- stool or stool culture on specialized selective culture media can be diagnostic.
- Food borne-botulism: stool, serum, vomits, gastric contents and suspected food should be collected to examine for spores or toxin.
- Hemorrhagic colitis caused by enterohemorrhagic E. coli can be detected by latex agglutination test.

Abuse of Drugs

The term 'drug abuse' connotes social disapproval. Any use of a drug for non-medical purposes, usually for altering consciousness but also for body building is known as abuse of drug. Psychological dependence (drug seeking behavior in which the individual uses the drug repetitively for personal satisfaction), physiologic dependence (withdrawal of the drug produces symptoms & signs), &tolerance (necessitating large doses of the drug to achieve the same response) are the main features of drugs of abuse. Some of the common drugs of abuse are discussed here.

a. Alcohols

Alcohol, primarily in the form of ethyl alcohol (ethanol), has occupied an important place in the history of human kind for at least 8000 years. Young children, chronic alcoholics or suicidal persons may ingest toxic quantities of one or several of the alcohols. Whether intentional or accidental, alcohol ingestions remain one of the more common, yet potentially devastating, poisonings commonly encountered in the emergency department. Ethanol is mildly polar and readily penetrates cell membrane. Approximately 25% of ingested ethanol is absorbed unaltered from the stomach and the rest from the small intestine. Distribution is rapid and wide. Over 90% of alcohol consumed is oxidized in the liver; much of the remainder is excreted through the lungs and in the urine. Alcohol is a central nervous system depressant. It can cause sedation, impaired motor function, slurred speech, emesis, ataxia etc. At high blood concentrations, it induces coma, respiratory depression, and death.

Laboratory analysis

Routine laboratory tests

CBC, electrolyte, BUN, glucose, creatinine, arterial blood gas analysis

Specific laboratory tests Qualitative test Specimen

Urine, stomach contents, scene residues.

Reagent

Potassium dichromate (25 g/1) in aqueous sulfuric acid (500 ml/1)

Procedure

1. Apply 50 µl of potassium dichromate solution to a strip of glass- fibre filter- paper and insert the paper in the neck of a test- tube containing 1 ml of sample.
2. Lightly stopper the tube and place in a boiling water-bath for 2 minutes.

Results

A change in colour from orange to green indicates the presence of volatile reducing agents such as ethanol; metaldehyde, methanol and paraldehyde.

Sensitivity

Ethanol, 0.5 g/1

Quantitative assay

Specimen

Whole blood, plasma, or serum (0.5 ml)

Reagents (see Annexure I)

1. Semicarbazide reagent.
2. Aqueous nicotinamide adenine dinucleotide (NAD) This solution is stable for 2-3 months at 4°C, but can be decomposed by vigorous agitation.
3. Alcohol dehydrogenase (ADH) suspension.
4. Aqueous perchloric acid

Standards

Solutions containing ethanol concentrations of 0.5, 1.0, 2.0 and 4.0 g/l prepared in heparinized whole blood to which 10 g/l sodium fluoride has been added. These solutions are stable for up to 1 month if stored at 4°C in well-sealed containers.

Procedure

1. Add 0.5 ml of blood to 2 ml of perchloric acid solution in a test- tube.
2. Vortex-mix for 30 seconds and then centrifuge for 5 minutes.
3. Add 0.1 ml of the supernatant (or 0.2 ml of an aqueous dilution (1:9) of plasma/serum) to a 10-ml tube containing 4.5 ml of semicarbazide reagent and vortex-mix for 10 seconds.
4. Add 0.1 ml of NAD solution and 0.02 ml of ADH suspension and mix gently so as not to cause foaming.
5. Allow to stand for 70 minutes at 20-25°C and measure the absorbance at 340 nm against a reagent blank.

Results

Construct a calibration graph of absorbance against blood ethanol concentration by analysis of the standard ethanol solutions and calculate the concentration of ethanol in the sample.

N.B. -If the specimen contains an ethanol concentration of more than 4.0 g/l, the analysis should be repeated using a dilution (1:1 or 1:3) of the sample in blank plasma. Methanol does not interfere, but propan-2-ol and some higher alcohols will reduce NAD under the conditions used in this assay.

- In all cases where the analysis may be delayed, it is important to add 10 g/l sodium fluoride to the specimen to inhibit microbial bio-transformation.

Sensitivity

Ethanol, 0.5 g/l

Treatment

Symptomatic management

Gastric lavage

Hemodialysis

In chronic toxicity thiamine can be given

b. Nicotine toxicity

Nicotine is one of the most widely abused chemical and now considered to be one of the most addicting substances. It is the principal pharmacologically active component of tobacco in which poisoning may occur in accidental ingestions of tobacco products (especially by children), use of nicotine-containing gums, and industrial exposure to tobacco products, contact with some pesticides and so on.

Nicotine has both stimulant and depressant action. Nicotine is readily absorbed through intact skin as well as through mucus membranes and the respiratory tract. It is metabolized by the liver and excreted by the kidney. Victims can complain of nausea, emesis, excessive salivation, and diarrhea at low doses. But at high dose it can cause respiratory paralysis, cardiovascular collapse, and convulsions.

There is no simple qualitative test for Nicotine, but this compound can be detected and identified by thin layer chromatography of a basic solvent extract of urine.

Laboratory analysis

General test

CBC (polymorph nuclear leukocytosis), electrolytes, BUN, creatinine, arterial blood-gas analysis, liver function tests, urine analysis (Glycosuria)

Toxin specific tests

- Serum nicotine levels should be determined as early as possible, but the short half-life of nicotine makes it difficult to accurately assess the level of intoxication.
- Urine nicotine levels – are inconsistent owing to the altered excretion of nicotine with changes in urine pH. They may be useful as a guide to the level of chronic exposures.

C. Opioids

Opioids comprise a broad spectrum of substances that include opiate alkaloids (e.g., morphine & codeine), synthetic opioids (e.g. pethidine) & semi synthetic opioids (e.g. heroin). They exert their effect acting on opiate receptors located within the CNS resulting in analgesia & euphoria. Opioids are used to treat cough, diarrhea, dyspnea (congestive heart failure), and sometimes anxiety as well as pain. The most commonly abused drugs in this group are heroin, and morphine. Tolerance and dependence of opioids develop with chronic use. The classic triad for opioid poisoning is miosis, coma and respiratory depression.

Laboratory analysis

General tests

Arterial blood gas analysis (ABGs), CBC, electrolytes, BUN, creatinine and blood glucose measurements in victims with abnormal vital signs or mental status.

Toxic-specific tests

Quantitative opioid blood levels are not clinically useful. Qualitative analysis (screening) of the urine by thin-layer chromatography can detect some but not all opioids. Gas chromatography and enzyme-linked immunoassays or radioimmunoassay are more sensitive for detecting specific agents. Confirming the presence of a specific opioid is not necessary when the history and response to antidote (naloxone) are consistent with a generic diagnosis of opioid poisoning.

Specific laboratory tests

Qualitative test

The Quick Screen One-Step Rapid Opiates Test technology (screen test for Morphine, Heroin, Codeine, &opium) incorporates a chromatographic absorbent device in which the drug or drug metabolites in the sample compete with an opiates derivative immobilized on a porous membrane for limited antibody sites. This is the preferred method for qualitative assay.

In the assay procedure, urine mixes with labeled antibody-dye conjugate and migrates through test device. When opiates levels are below 2000 mg/ml (the detection cutoff sensitivity of the test) unbound antibody-dye conjugate binds to immobilized antigen conjugate in the Test Zone (T), producing a pink-rose colored band that indicates a negative result. Conversely, when opiates levels are above the detection limit, antibody-dye conjugate binds to the free drug, forming an antigen-antibody-dye complex. The complex competes with immobilized antigen conjugate in the Test Zone, preventing the development of a pink-rose colored band. Regardless of the test result, a color band is produced in the Control Zone (C) by a non-specific sandwich dye conjugate reaction. This band serves as a built-in quality

Specimen

Urine

Procedure

1. Collect a urine sample from test subject using a suitable clean container preferably glass.
2. Refrigerated specimens or other materials should be equilibrated to room temperature before testing.
3. Open the foil pouch at the notch, remove the test device, and label the device with specimen ID.
4. Holding the dropper vertically, add four drops of urine into the sample well 'S' waiting 5 seconds between drops.
5. Observe migration or lateral flow of the sample across the entire test panel. Add additional sample drops if migration is not complete.

6. Positive results may be observed as soon as 5 minutes, depending on the concentration of opiates in the tested specimen. To confirm negative results, a complete reaction time of 8-10 minutes is required. Do not interpret results after 15 minutes.

Results

Positive: One pink rose band appears in the control zone and no band appears in the test zone. A positive result indicates the opiates level is 2000ng/ml or higher in the test urine sample. Negative: One band appears in the test zone and other band appears in the control zone. A negative result indicates that the opiates level is below the detection sensitivity of 2000ng/ml.

N.B. any line, no matter how faint appearing in the test area confirms a negative test.

Invalid: If there are no distinct color bands visible in both the test zone and the control zone or if there is a visible band in the test zone but not in the control zone, then the test is invalid. In the instant, retesting of the specimen is recommended.

Natural Toxicants

Natural substances are also still occasionally featured in accidental poisoning cases, when compared to poisoning by others. Many plants & animals produce toxic substances for both defense & offensive purposes. Natural toxins may feature in poisoning via containing in food, by accidental ingestions of poisonous plants or animals & by stinging & biting. Natural toxins are of diverse structure & mode of action, & there are far too many categories to cover in this short topic. So we like to give an overview on it.

a. Animal toxins

Animal toxins comprise a diverse range of structures & modes of action. A simple & well known example is formic acid which is found in ants. Animal toxins are often mixtures of complex proteins. Most of us suffer from animal toxins at some time in our lives. However, in some countries death & illness due to animal poisons represents a significant proportion of cases.

Snake venom

Snake bite is one of the most common forms of poisoning by natural toxins worldwide. The snake venom is a complex mixture of compounds. The enzymatic components of snake venom cause local and sometimes systemic effects, and the non-enzymatic components provide lethality. Absorption of snake venom is variable but most rapid through the blood vessels. Distribution depends on protein binding, membrane permeability and pH. The kidney excretes venom. Clinical presentations of snakebite may be obvious, but not always. It can cause anaphylactic reactions, nausea, vomiting, diarrhea, hemolytic anemia, hemorrhage, respiratory failure.

Laboratory tests

- Basic studies should be performed: CBC; platelet count; coagulation tests; electrolytes, creatinine and BUN levels.
- Urinalysis initially and with subsequent bedside checks using dip sticks can signal developing hematuria or myoglobinuria.
- Attempts to develop assays that identify the presence of venom at the puncture site or within the victim's serum have met with little success. A radioimmunoassay was developed for this purpose, but it has never become a practical methodology and is useful only as a research tool. The enzyme-linked immunmosorbant assay bridges the gap because it can detect small amounts of antigen antibody complex.

Treatment

- Incision & suction (source of controversy because of tissue damage & it is better to use with a vacuum pump)
- Antivenoms (definitive)

b. Plant toxins

Many species of plants contain toxic chemicals. There are many well known plant toxins ranging from the irritant formic acid found in nettles to more poisonous compounds such as atropine (atropa belladonna). The concentration of toxic chemicals is variable among the same species & different species.

Major toxic effects are on the skin (e. g allergic dermatitis), GIT (e. g., gastroenteritis), cardiovascular (e .g., arrhythmia).

Annexure I

Preparation of Reagents

1. Reagents for lead qualitative tests

a. Sodium tartrate buffer, pH 2.8.

Sodium bitartate	19 g
Tartaric acid	15 g
purified water	1000ml
PH	2.8

b. Aqueous sodium rhodizonate solution (10 g/l).

2. Reagents preparation for quantitative tests of lead using AAS

a. Nitric acid- Sub-boiling redistilled ultra-pure concentrated nitric acid is required to prepare the reagents.

b. Diluent- The diluent (and matrix modifier) is 10.0 mL/L Triton X-100 and 2.0-g/L ammonium dihydrogen phosphate in 0.2% nitric acid.

c. Calibrators- The calibrators are prepared from a stock reference solution containing lead at 1000 µg/mL, and then diluted further with diluent to achieve final concentrations of 10, 20, 40, and 60 µg/dl, which are used to calibrate the instrument as described below.

d. Controls- The control material is a commercial whole blood control.

3. Thin layer preparation for organophosphorus insecticides

a. Reconstitute the extract in 100 µl of methanol and spot 20 µl on a column marked on the plate.

b. Spot 10 µl of the standard mixture on a second column.

c. Develop the chromatogram (10-cm run) using cyclohexane: acetone: chloroform (saturated tank) and allow to dry.

d. Spray the plate with 4-(p-nitrobenzyl) pyridine solution and heat, preferably in an oven, at 110°C for 30 minutes.

e. Allow to cool and spray with acetone: tetraethylenepentamine (9:1).

4. Reagent preparation in the qualitative test of aspirin

Trinder's reagent- Mix 40 g of mercuric chloride dissolved in 850 ml of purified water with 120 ml of aqueous hydrochloric acid (1mol/1) and 40 g of hydrated ferric nitrate, and dilute to 1 liter with purified water.

5. Reagent preparation for quantitative assay of barbiturates

a. Borate buffer, pH 8.4. Mix 22.4 g of disodium tetraborate with 76 ml of aqueous hydrochloric acid (1 mol/1) and dilute to 2 liters with purified water.

B. Aqueous hydrochloric acid (2 mol /1).

c. Concentrated sulfuric acid (relative density 1.83).

d. Concentrated ammonium hydroxide (relative density 0.88). w. Sodium sulfate/charcoal mixture. Add 100 mg of activated charcoal to 100 g of anhydrous sodium sulfate, mix thoroughly and heat in an evaporating basin at 100°C for 8 hours. Allow to cool and store in a tightly stoppered bottle.

Standard solution preparation for qualitative assay of barbiturates Solutions containing barbital at concentrations of 5, 10, 25 and 50 mg/1 in blank human plasma, prepared by dilution from an aqueous solution of barbital sodium (1.12 g/1), equivalent to diethylbarbituric acid at a concentration of 1.00 g/1.

6. Reagent preparation for cholinesterase activity test

a. Dithiobisnitrobenzoate reagent. 5, 5'-Dithiobis (2-nitrobenzoic add) (0.2 g/1) in sodium dihydrogen orthophosphate buffer (0.1 mol/1, pH 7.4).

b. Aqueous acetylthiocholine iodide solution (5 g/1).

c. Aqueous pralidoxime chloride solution (200 g/l).

d. Plasma or serum from an unexposed individual (control plasma).

7. Reagent preparation for qualitative test of acetaminophen

a. Saturated o-cresol- Mix 10 mL of o-cresol with 1 L of deionized water. Allow to stand for 24 h before use. Solution will be stable for 1 year at room temperature.

b. Ammonium hydroxid, 4 mol /L - Dilute 284 mL of concentrated ammonium hydroxide to 1 L with deionized water. Solution will be stable for 1 year at room temperature.

c. Concentrated hydrochloric acid.

8. Reagents preparations for quantitative test of Acetaminophen

a. Acetaminophen stock reference solution, 1000 mg/L - Dissolve 100 mg of acetaminophen in 20 mL of methanol and then dilute to 100mL with deionized water. Solution is stable for at least 6 months when stored refrigerated.

b. Calibrator - Dilute the acetaminophen stock reference solution with deionized water to provide working calibrators of 20 and 100 µg/mL. Calibrators are stable for 2 months when stored refrigerated.

c. 3-Acetamidophenol stock internal standard, 1000 mg/L - Dissolve 100 mg of 3-acetamidophenol in 20 mL of methanol and dilute to 100 mL with deionized water. Solution is stable for 6 months when stored refrigerated.

d. 3-Acetaminophen working internal standard, 50 mg/ml. Dilute 5 mL of the stock internal standard to 100 mL with deionized water. Solution is stable for 2 months when stored refrigerated.

e. Phosphate buffer, 0.225 mol/l, pH 7.4 - Mix 80.4 ml of disodium hydrogen phosphate (Na2HPO4) solution (30.6 g/ l) with 19.6 ml of potassium dihydrogen phosphate (KH2PO4) solution (31.9 g/l). Adjust to pH 7.4, if necessary, with the appropriate phosphate solution. Solution is stable for 2 months when stored at room temperature.

f. Mobile phase: sodium acetate buffer/acetonitrile (92/8) by volume) - Add 80 ml of acetonitrile to a 1 lt volumetric flask and dilute to volume with 0.01 mol/1 sodium acetate buffer, pH 4.0. Filter through a 0.5-µm pore-size filter and degas by applying gentile vacuum.

9. Reagents for quantitative test of ethanol.

a. Semicarbazide reagent.

Tetrasodium pyrophosphate dehydrated	10 g.
Semicarbazide hydrochloride	2.5 g
Glycine	0.5 g
Distilled water	250 ml
Sodium hydroxide (2 mol/l)	10ml

Dilute the solution by Distilled water up to 300ml

b. Aqueous nicotinamide adenine dinucleotide (NAD) This solution is stable for 2-3 months at 4°C, but can be decomposed by vigorous agitation.

c. Alcohol dehydrogenase (ADH) suspension

Ammonium sulfate	45.5 g
Tetra sodium pyrophosphate (dehydrated)	3 g
Distilled water	100 ml
Crystalline yeast ADH	2.5 g

Adjust pH to 7.3 with either aqueous hydrochloric acid or sodium hydroxide (both1 mol/l) this solution is stable for 2-3 months at 4°C.

d. Aqueous perchloric acid

Perchloric acid (700 ml/l)	2.9 ml
Distilled water	100 ml

Annexure II

Apparatuses

1. *Atomic Absorption spectrophotometer for quantitative analysis of Lead*

A good-quality graphite furnace atomic absorption spectrometer is required for analysis. The graphite furnace requires a L'vov platform to give optimal sensitivity and accuracy. Zeeman's background correction is useful to reduce the effect of background to a minimum.

2. *Supplies for spectrophotometer for quantitative analysis of Lead*

Polypropylene pipette tips, specimen cups, and Teflon reagent storage bottles are required. Before use, they are leached in 10% nitric acid for 1 week and rinsed in triple- distilled water.

3. *HPLC equipment for quantitative test of Acetaminophen*

A 250 x 4.5-mm –I.D. column containing octadecylsilane (C18) bonded-silica particles (5-µm diameter) is used for the analysis of acetaminophen. The HPLC system is equipped with a fixed-(254-nm) or variable-wavelength detector set at a sensitivity of 0.1 or 0.2 absorbance units full scale for acetaminophen concentrations of 0 to 200 or 200 to 500-µg/ml, respectively. The pump flow rate is 1.5 ml/min.

4. *Summary of basic equipment required for toxicological analyses*

Reliable, regularly serviced and calibrated laboratory balances

Bench-top centrifuge (electrical or hand-driven) for separating blood samples and solvent extracts

Vortex-mixer or other form of mechanical or hand-driven

shaker such as a rotary mixer

Water-bath and (electrical) heating block

Spirit lamp or butane gas burner

Refrigerator (electrical or evaporative) for storing standards/ samples

PH meter

Range of automatic and semi-automatic pipettes

Low-power, polarizing microscope

An adequate supply of laboratory glassware, including volumetric apparatus, and adequate cleaning facilities

A supply of chemically pure water

A supply of compressed air or nitrogen

A supply of thin-layer chromatography plates or facilities for preparing such plates

Facilities for developing and visualizing thin-layer chromatograms, including an ultraviolet lamp (254 nm and 366 nm) and a fume cupboard or hood

Single-beam or dual-beam ultraviolet/visible spectrophotometer and associated cells

Conway microdiffusion apparatus

Porcelain spotting tile

Modified Gutzeit apparatus

Annexure III

Glossary of Terms

Abuse- Excessive or improper use of drugs or other substances.

Acetylcholine- the main neurotransmitter of the vertebrate and invertebrate in the peripheral nervous systems

Acetylcholinesterase- enzyme that hydrolyses the neurotransmitter acetylcholine.

Acidosis- Pathological condition resulting from accumulation of acid in, or loss of base from, the blood or body tissues.

Acute- Sudden or short-term.

Anemia- Deficiency of erythrocytes or of hemoglobin in the blood.

Antibody- A protein produced in the body in response to exposure to an antigen; it recognizes and specifically binds the antigen.

Anticoagulant- A drug that prevents clotting of blood.

Antidote- An agent that neutralizes or opposes the action of a poison on an organism.

Arrhythmia (dysrhythmia)- Any variation from the normal rhythm of the heartbeat.

Antigen- Any substance that stimulates the body to produce an antibody.

Bilirubin- A pigment, derived from the breakdown of hemoglobin that occurs in soluble form in blood and in bile.

Blank- Used in analytical chemistry to denote a specimen not containing the analyte of interest and from which a background reading can be obtained.

Carboxyhaemoglobin- Product formed when carbon monoxide binds to hemoglobin.

Chelate- Compound in which a central metallic ion is attached to an organic molecule (chelating agent) at two or more positions

Chelating agent- A compound capable of forming a chelate with a metal ion.

Cholinesterase- Enzyme that catalysis the breakdown of a choline ester to choline (see also: Acetylcholinesterase).

Chronic- Long-term (cf. Acute).

Contaminant- An impurity.

Corrosive- Able to eat away or dissolve by chemical action.

Cosmetic- Concerned with improving appearance or hygiene.

Cross-contamination- Accidental introduction of an impurity.

Crystalluria- Presence of crystals in the urine.

Cutaneous- Associated with the skin.

Cyanosis- Blue appearance, especially of the skin and mucous membranes, due to deficient oxygenation.

Dermal- Relating to the skin.

Detergent- A chemical cleaning agent.

Diuresis- Increased production of urine.

Diuresis, forced- Abnormally enhanced urine production, for example following administration of intravenous fluids or diuretics.

Drug- A substance that, when administered to an organism or a system derived from an organism, may modify one or more of its functions.

Emesis- Vomiting.

Emetic- Substance causing emesis.

Erythrocyte- Red blood cell.

Fumigant- A vapour used to kill pests.

Fungicide- A pesticide used to kill fungi or check the growth of spores.

Haematocrit- Erythrocyte volume fraction; the ratio by volume of the blood cells to plasma.

Haematuria- presence of red blood cells in the urine.

Haemodialysis- Procedure whereby blood is dialysed against a large volume of isotonic fluid outside the body and then returned to the systemic circulation. Used to remove unwanted compounds of low relative molecular mass from the circulation.

Haemoglobin- An iron-containing pigment found in erythrocytes, which binds oxygen for transport within the bloodstream.

Haemolysis- Rupture of erythrocytes leading to the appearance of free haemoglobin in the plasma.

Herbicide- A pesticide used to control or kill plants or plant seeds.

Hydrolysis- Decomposition caused by or involving water.

Hyperglycaemia- Abnormally high blood sugar (glucose) concentration.

Hyperventilation- Increased rate and depth of respiration

Hypoglycaemia- Abnormally low blood sugar (glucose) concentration.

Hypostatic- caused by the combined effects of gravity & poor circulation of the blood.

Hypoxia- Reduction of oxygen in an animal body below physiological requirements.

Metabolic acidosis- Acidosis of metabolic origin.

Metabolite- A substance produced by biotransformation.

Methaemoglobin- Oxidized haemoglobin.

Miosis- Contraction of the pupil of the eye.

Mixer, rotar- A device for mixing solutions or suspensions by means of a gentle rotating motion. Used for solvent extraction or other procedures requiring mixing of relatively large quantities of material.

Opiate- A pharmacologically active agent, such as morphine, derived from opium.

Osmolality- The osmotic strength of a solution.

Pesticide- Substance used to kill or control any pest, including animals, plants, fungi, or other organisms in agricultural, industrial and domestic situations

Pipette, automatic- Device used to dispense repeatedly known volumes of a fluid.

Pipette, positive-displacement- Device with a washable tip, used to take up and dispense known volumes of a fluid, and in which the plunger is in contact with the fluid. Used to dispense viscous solutions such as whole blood.

Pipette, semi-automatic- Device, often with disposable tips, used to take up and dispense known volumes of aqueous fluids such as plasma or serum. Reliable only for fluids with a viscosity similar to that of water.

Scene residue- Material found at the scene of a poisoning incident.

Supernatant - An upper layer of liquid.

Tolerance- (i) The ability of an organism to experience exposure to potentially harmful amounts of a poison without showing evidence of toxicity. (ii) An adaptive state whereby the pharmacological effects of the same dose of a substance become diminished as a result of repeated exposure.

Toxic- Able to cause injury to living organisms as a result of chemical interaction within the organism.

Relative volume of distribution- is volume of distribution divided by body weight.

Respiratory acidosis- Acidosis of respiratory origin.

Vortex-mixer- A device for mixing solutions or suspensions by means of a whirling motion which creates a cavity in the centre of the mixture. Used for solvent extraction and other procedures requiring efficient mixing of relatively small quantities of material (up to about 10 ml total volume).

Xenobiotic- Compound foreign to the biotransformation of an organism.

Annexure IV

Abbreviations Used

AAS- Atomic absorption spectroscopy

ABGs- Arterial blood gas analysis

ALA- D- Delta amino levulinate dehydratase

BUN- Blood urea &nitrogen

CBC- Complete blood count

CNS- Central nervous system

CO- Carbon monoxide

DDT- Dichloro-Diphenyl-Trichloroethane

EPP- Erythrocyte proto porphyrine

GC- Gas chromatography

GC-MS- Gas chromatography-Mass spectrometry

GIT- Gastrointestinal tract

HCl- Hydrochloric acid

HPLC- High performance liquid chromatography

NaOH- Sodium hydroxide nm- nano meter

NMR- Nuclear magnetic resonance

PH- Power of hydrogen

PT- Prothrombin time

PTT- Partial prothrombin time t1/2 - Half-life

TLC- Thin layer chromatography

UV- Ultraviolet

Vd- Volume of distribution

Bibliography

1. Woodroffmand Amie Ali, *Law of Evidence*, (1979) 14 th Edn.
2. L.A. Lyons, *Medical Jurisprudence for India*, 5 th Edn.1914.
3. Allen, Michael, *Textbook on Criminal Law*, 7 th ed., Oxford University Press, 2003.
4. Basu's *Indian Penal Code*, 9th ed, 2006.
5. Srivastava, R.C., *Law Relating to Crime and Punishment*, 2006, Manav Law House, Allahabad, 2006.
6. Pillai, K.N. Chandrasekharan, *General Principles of Criminal Law*, 1st Ed., reprint, Eastern Book Company, Lucknow, 2005.
7. *The Penal Law of India*, Vol. 1, 11 th ed., Law Publishers (India) Pvt. Ltd., Allahabad, 2002.
8. Dempsey, John S. (2007), *Introduction to Investigation*, Second Edition, Florida, USA: CRC Press.
9. Encyclopedia Britannica (1994), The New Encyclopedia Britannica: Knowledge in Depth, *Macropaedia*, Volume 21, New York, USA: Encyclopedia Britanica.
10. James, Stuart C., Joft J. Nordby and Suzanne S. Bell (2009), *Forensic Science: An Introduction to Scientific and Investigative Techniques*, Third Edition, California, USA: CRC Press.
11. Genard, Dorothy A. (2007), *Forensic Entomology: An Introduction*, California, USA: John Wiley & Sons Ltd.
12. Lyde, D.P. (2004), *Forensics for Dummies*, Indiana, USA: West Publishing, Inc.
13. Timmermans, Stefan S. (2007), *Postmortem: How Medical Examiners Explain Suspicious Deaths*, Chicago, USA: University of Chicago Press.

14. Waters, Brenda L., Editor (2004), *Handbook of Autopsy Practice*, 4th Edition, Ohio, USA: Humana Press.

15. Websters, Ralph Waldo A. (2000), *Legal Medicine and Toxicology*, California, USA: W.B. Saunders Publishing.

16. Suzanne Bell, *Encyclopedia of Forensic Science*, Facts On File, Inc., NY, 2008.

17. Richard Shepherd, *Simpson's Forensic Medicine*, Twelfth Edition, Arnold, U.K., 2003.

18. Blackwood, Alexander Leslie, *A Manual of Materia Medica, Therapeutics and Pharmacology*, Boericke & Tafel, Philadelphia, 1906.

19. Peter Viccellio, MD, *Hand book of Medical Toxicology*, First edition, 1993.

20. B. Widdop, F.A. & de Wolff, R.A. Braithwaite, R.J. Flanagan, S.S. Brown, *Basic Analytical Toxicology*, 1995, WHO.

21. Katzung B.G., *Basic and Clinical Pharmacology*, 8th edition, 2001.

22. Carl A.B, &Edward R.A, *Teitz Textbook of clinical chemistry*, 3rd edition, 1999.

23. Eyasu Mekonon., *Pharmacology for Medical Students*, vol. II, 2nd edition, Addis Ababa, 1999.

24. P.D Sharma, *Environmental Biology and Toxicology*, secondary edition, 2002-2003.

25. Philip C. Burcham, *An Introduction to Toxicology*, Springer, 1st edn., 2014.

26. Lindsay Murray, *Toxicology Handbook*, 3rd Edition, Elsevier, 2015.

27. Nicholas T Lappas, *Forensic Toxicology: Principles and Concepts*, Academic Press, 1 st Edn., 2016.

Notes on Spagyrics

By Dr. Debasish Kundu

Rs. 395/- US $ 21.50 Paperback

In this book author briefly discusses the principles of Alchemy with some exceptional notes on Sexual and Spiritual Alchemy.

CONTENTS: Note to the Readers, Foreword, Preface, Introduction, History of Alchemy, Spagyrics, Principles of Spagyrics, The Quest for the Quintessence, Plant Alchemy, Energetic Spagyrics, The Three Philosophical Principles, Spagyric Electro-Homoeopathy, Energy in the Organism, Herbal Medicine, Spiritual Alchemy, Sexual Alchemy, Spagyric Meditation, Hermetic Philosophy, Fermentation and Distillation of Wine Spirit, Spagyric Experiments, Explanation of Some Spagyrics Terms, Bibliography

Materia Medica and Practice of Medicine in Electro-Homoeopathy

By Dr.Debasish Kundu

Rs. 395/- US $ 21.50 Paperback

CONTENTS: Foreword, Preface, Electrohomoeopathy-An Introduction, Life History of Count Cesare Mattei, Preparation of Electro Homoeopathic Remedies, Electrohomoeopathy Formulas, Constitution and Temperament, Materia Medica of Electrohomoeopathy Medicines, Examination of the Patient, General Rules for Using the Medicines, Practice of Medicine, Points for External Application, Chief Points and their Uses, Clinical Index, Bibliography

Treatise on Spagyric Homoeopathic Pharmacy

By Dr. Debasish Kundu & Dr. Vijay Kant Agnihotri, Sr. Scientist, CSIR, Foreworded By Prof. Raffaele Pezzani, University of Padova, Italy

Rs. 395/- US $ 21.50 Paperback

It features all necessary information about the method of preparations and formulations of Zimpel, Krauss and Bernus. It is the only book which has incorporated Spagyrics formulas of Zimpel brought back from the lost fragments of time.

According to Prof. Pezzani, it is definitely a valuable guide, a friend that every Electrohomeopathy (according to Mattei) practitioner should possess. It is a must have collection for everyone.

CONTENTS: Dedication, Foreword, Preface, Spagyric Homeopathic Pharmacy, Electrohomoeopathy Formulas, Spagyrics after Zimpel, Krauss and Bernus, Medicinal Plants, Tables of Essential Oil Yielding Plants, Bibliography

Materia Medica for the New Age Man

By Dr. Debasish Kundu, Dr A.Jayasuriya, Chancellor, The Open International University, Colombo and Edited by Dr. M Ahmed, Member, Bangladesh Homeopathy Board, Dhaka

Rs. 450/- US $ 24.50 Hardbound

This is the only book which covered all therapeutic schools of Homeopathy, from Gemmotherapy, Lithotherapy, Bach flower to Spagyric Homeopathy.

CONTENTS: Foreword to the Second Edition, Introduction, Introduction to Homeopathy, Evolution of Disease, Introduction to Vital Force, Miasms, Homeopathic Pharmacy, Case Taking, Doctrine of Dosage, Therapeutic Schools of Homeotherapeutics at a Glance, Nosodes and Sarcodes, Materia Medica, Clinical Index of Homeopathic Remedies, Mother Tinctures (External Use), Do's and Don'ts for Patients, Clinical Tips for Dummies, General Index of Remedies, References

Treatise on Electro-Homoeopathic Pharmacy

By Dr. Debasish Kundu & Dr.Ajit Singh, Forewarded By Prof. Fabio R Ambrosi, Chairman, Mattei Archieves, Italy

Rs. 195/- US $ 15.50 Paperback

CONTENTS: Foreword, Preface, Introduction to Electro Homoeopathic Pharmacy, Laboratory Equipments Used in Electro Homoeopathy Pharmacy, Vehicles used in Electrohomoeopathy, Sources of Electro Homoeopthic Medicines, Collection of Medicinal Plants, Cohobation: An Extraordinary Pharmacy, Methods of Preparation of Spagyric Medicines, Quality Control Procedures, Pharmacodynamics of Electrohomoeopathy Essences, Dosages and Mode of Administration, List of Medicinal Plants Used in

Electrohomoeopathic Remedies, Appendix 1: Terminology, Appendix 2: Prescription Writing, Appendix 3: Biographies, Appendix 4: Apparatus, Bibliography

Essentials of Acupuncture

By Dr. Debasish Kundu & Prof. Choo Led Sin, Chairman, International Federation of Acupuncture, Singapore

Rs. 995/- US $ 40.00 Hardbound

The Only Book which deals with Acupuncture Anaesthesia

CONTENTS: Preface, Introduction, History of Acupuncture, Philosophy of Acupuncture, Five Elements Theory, Diagnosis in Traditional Chinese Medicine, Evaluation and Diagnosis, The Concept of Qi, Management & Research on Some Disorders, How Acupuncture Works, Acupuncture Anesthesia, Laser Acupuncture, Auriculotherapy, Atlas of Acupuncture Points, Therapeutics of Common Ailments, Therapeutics of Common Ailments, Infertility, Impotence and Acupuncture, Acupuncture in Hairfall, Does Acupuncture Hurts, Related Therapies, Explanation of Some Terms, Marmapuncture, Bibliography

Cesare Mattei's Principles of Electro Homeopathy

Interpreted & Revised By Dr. Debasish Kundu

Rs. 395/- US $ 21.50 Paperback

The classic text has been Rewritten in simple language with much needed Interpretation & Revision. In some places the original French edition has been consulted, also enriched with footnotes wherever necessary.

CONTENTS: Preface by Editor, What is Electro-Homeopathy?, Names of the Electro-Homeopathic Remedies, General Information about the Electro-Homeopathic Remedies, Sphere of Action of the Remedies in Globules, General Remarks on the Electric Liquids, Their Mode of Application, Results of Experience, Doses and Method of Administration of the Remedies in Globules, Of Diagnosis, Principles and Rules for the Selection of the Appropriate Remedy, Easy Experiments for Beginners, Catalogue of Diseases Cured by Electro-Homeopathy, Appendix

Stepping Stones to Electo-Homoeopathy (Count Mattei's System of Medicine)

By A J L Gliddon(Original Edition with Vitiation of Blood and Lymph Theory)

Rs. 395/- US $ 21.50 Paperback

A brief insight into the discovery of electro homeopathy together with a rational explanation of the principles involved and the proposed medicines.

CONTENTS: Introduction , The Human Body, Count Mattei's Theories, Symptoms of Disease, The Electro-Homceopathic Remedies, The Globule Remedies, The Electricities, External Use of Electricities, External Use of Globules, Baths, Compresses, etc., How to Select the Remedies, How to Determine the Dose, Dilutions, Dry Globules, Table of Doses, Minute Doses, Effects of the Remedies, Other Hygienic Helps, Diet, Dress, Pure Air, etc.

Essentials of Trace Elements & Biochemic Medicine

By Prof. Dr. Debasish Kundu, Edited By Prof. Seyed Farzin Hassanzadeh Salehian Ph.D. (Iran)

Rs. 350/- US $ 19.00 Paperback

Cell Salts or Bioplasgens have always been considered an important part of healing in Homeopathy and Spagyrics. This book contains all essential materials concerning Trace Elements & Bioplasgen and their relationship with Spagyrics, Clinical Materia Medica with useful suggestions.

CONTENTS: Preface, Introduction to Trace Elements & Bioplasgens, The Functions of The Cell, Astrology and Bioplasgens, Minerals, Trace Elements, Materia Medica of the Bioplasgens, Bio-combinations, Bibliography

A Textbook on Food, Nutrition and Dietetics

By Dr. Debasish Kundu Editor Dr. Malik A.K. Awan Ph.D. (London), Associate Editor Prof. Seyed Farzin Hassanzadeh Salehian Ph.D.(Iran)

Rs. 495/- US $ 20.00 Paperback

CONTENTS: Preface, Relationship between Food, Nutrition & Health, History of Nutrition, Functions of Food, Digestion of Food, Food and Nutrition, Nutrition, Diet & Development, Nutrition & Diet Therapy, Nutrition for Infants, Children, Adults, Women and Elderly, Ideal Diet Plan, The Food Pyramid, Therapeutic Diet, Bibliography

Notes on MJT (Forensic Medicine & Toxicology)

By Dr. Debasish Kundu Ph.D. Assisted By Dr. Ravi Justin Raj NMD, LLB Edited By Dr. Malik A.K. Awan B.S., M.S. (Psychology), D.C.L., D.D. (U.S.A.), Ph.D. (London)

Rs. 550/- US $ 22.00 Paperback

CONTENTS: Part I: Forensic Medicine: Dedication , Preface , Introduction, Scope of Forensic Medicine, Aspects of Identification, Medico-legal Aspects of Death, Investigation of Death, Death by Asphyxia, Medico-legal Aspects of Injuries, Investigation of Wounds, Medico-legal Aspects of Sex Crimes, Medico-legal Aspects of Abortion, Forensic Pathology, Forensic Entomology, Radiation Poisoning, Medico-legal Sections in IPC, Cr PC, AND IE A, Part II: Toxicology: Introduction to Toxicology, General Approach to a Victim of Poison, Clinical Toxicology Laboratory, Practical Aspects of Analytical Toxicology, Toxicants of Public Health Hazard, Medical Toxicants, Environmental Toxicants, Abuse of Drugs, Natural Toxicants, Annexure I: Preparations of Reagents, Annexure II: Apparatuses, Annexure III: Glossary of Terms Used, Annexure IV: Abbreviations Used, Bibliography

Notes on Minor Surgery

By Dr. Debasish Kundu Ph.D. Guided & Edited by Dr. A.K. Banerjee M.B.B.S., M.D. (U.S.A.)

Rs. 395/- US $ 21.50 Paperback

CONTENTS: Part-I: Preface, Acharya Sushruta, Basic Surgical Procedures, Surgery of Some Common Conditions, Part II: Sterilisation, Suture Materials, Nomenclature of Operations, Planning for Operation, Anaesthesia,Operative Surgery, Postoperative Complications, Abscess Drainage, Venesection (Cut Down), Skin Grafting, Circumcision, Vasectomy, Hyderocele, Inguinal Hernia, Strangulated Inguinal Hernia, Femoral Hernia, Umbilical Hernia, Appendicetomy,

Abdominal Incisions, Peptic Ulcer, Vagotomy, Gastrojejumnostomy, Partial Gastrectomy, Closure of Perforated Peptic Ulcer, Right Hemicolectomy, Colostomy, Cholecystectomy, Choledocholithotomy (Supraduodenal), Spleenectomy, Lumbar Sympathectomy, Haemorrhoidectomy, Suprapubic Cystostomy, Prostatectomy, Exposure of Kidney , Exposure of the Ureter and Ureterolithotomy, Mastectomy, Thyroidectomy, Tracheostomy, Empyema Thoracis, Amputations, Bibliography

Principles and Practice of Naturopathy

By Dr. Debasish Kundu Editor Dr. Malik A. K. Awan Ph.D. (London) Associate Editor Prof. Sayed Farzin Hassanzadeh Salehian Ph.D.(Iran)

Rs. 750/- US $ 30.00 Paperback

CONTENTS: Foreword, Preface to the First Edition, Preface to the Third Edition, Naturopathy: Its Principles & Pioneers, Physiology, Food and Nutrition, Hygiene and Sanitation, Biology, Herbology, Medicinal Plants, Magnet Therapy, Yoga and Meditation, Massage Therapy, Medical Gymnastics, Chemistry, Bacteriology, Toxicology, Pathology, Osteology, Neurology, Ethics, Hydro Therapy and Helio Therapy, Colour Therapy, Fasting and Diet, Mud Therapy and Fango Therapy, Acupressure, Aromatherapy, Reflexology, Iridology, Vitamins and Balanced Diets, Bibliography

Diseases of Women (Adopted from Margaret Seifert's Krankheiten Der Franen)

By Dr. Shefalika Kundu, Edited By Dr. Debasish Kundu & Dr. Sudeshna Kundu

Rs. 350/- US $ 19.00 Paperback

The book is intended as a handbook on diseases of women with their Electrohomeopathic treatment. Besides an update on the literature on Contraception using Spagyrics , entirely new topics Anatomy of Uterus and Stages of development in Pregnancy are added.

CONTENTS: Preface to the Second Edition, Foreword to the First Edition, Preface, Introduction, Anatomy and Physiology of Sexual Organs of Women, General View of Treatment, Diseases and Their Treatment, Hygienic Care of the Body and Toilet, Anatomy of Uterus in Pregnancy, Notes on Various Diseases, Family Planning, Contraception in Electrohomoeopathy,Diet, Index of Diseases Discussed, Bibliography

Lectures on Materia Medica & Therapeutics

By Dr. H. D. Banerjee, Foreworded By M V Mattei, Thoroughly Revised & Edited By Prof. Dr. Debasish Kundu

Rs. 225/- US $ 18.00 Paperback

CONTENTS: Preface to the Third Edition, Preface to the Second Edition, Foreword to the First Edition, Introduction, On Electro-Homoeopathic Principles, On Principles of Orthodox School, On Homeopathic Principles , On Objections to Electro-Homoeopathy, Chemical Analysis of the Remedies, Dynamisation of the Remedies, On Minute Doses, On Frequency of the Doses, Purgatives in Electro-Homoeopathy, On Prescription Writing, Materia Medica & Therapeutics, On Therapeutics of the Remedies

Principles & Art of Cure in Electrohomeopathy

By Prof. Dr.Debasish Kundu Ph.D.

Rs. 195/- US $ 15.00 Paperback

CONTENTS: Introduction to Electrohomeopathy, Philosophy, The Discoverer, Principles of Nature, Introduction to Electrohomeopathy Medicines, The Iris science, Sources and preparation of Electrohomeopathy Medicines, Cohobation, Spagyric Tinctures, Classification of Electrohomeopathy Medicines, Classification, Preparation and Therapeutics uses of Electrohomeopathy Medicines, Potentisation of Electrohomeopathy Medicines and Electric fluids, Preparation and Therapeutic uses of Ointments and Lotions, Points for application Electric Fluids, Ointments and Lotions, Plain talks on using the medicines, Potentisation and Bio-Magnetism, The Similia of Electrohomeopathy, The Scientific basis of Electrohomeopathy System of Medicine, World's present day need of Electrohomeopathy, Clinical Index.

A Clinical Treatise on Cancer

By Prof. Dr.Debasish Kundu Ph.D. Foreworded By Dr. B.B. Upreti, Ph. D. General Secretary, All Nepal Electro-Homeo Medical Association, Hetauda, Nepal

Rs. 195/- US $ 15.00 Paperback

CONTENTS: Introduction, The Increase of Cancer and it's Causes, The Treatment of Cancer, Diet for Patients, Hygienic Care of the Patients

Books Published By LBO Publishing, 700 N Valley St., Suite B PMB 11884 Anaheim, CA 92801, USA Marketed In India Exclusively By Originals, Delhi

CONTENTS: Foreword, Preface, Part 1: Introduction to Spagyric Medicine, History of Alchemy, Principles of Spagyrics, The Simila of Alchemy, Difference Between Homoeopathy and Spagyric Homoeopathy, Botanical Consciousness in Spagyrics, Micronutrients and Spagyrics, Alchemy and the Zodiac Connection, How Spagyric Medicines Work, Alchemy and Spagyrics, Spagyrics : The Future in Medicine, Part 2: Pharmacy in Plant Alchemy, Pharmaceutical Process, Laboratory Apparatus, Vehicles Used in Plant Alchemy, Sources of Medicines, Preparation of Spagyric Essence, Spagyric Essence by Cohobation Method, Phytochemical Analysis of Plants, Different Spagyric Methods, Quality Control Procedures, Safety Measures in Laboratory, Doctrine of Dosage, Medicinal Plants, Terminology, Appendix, Bibliography

Mysticism, Romance & Secrets of Count Cesare Mattei (With Properly Transcripted Secret Formulas)

By Prof. Dr. Debasish Kundu , Ph.D. (U.S.A.)

Printed on Art Paper, USD ($) 40.00 Hard Bound

It is the Bible of Mattei Electrohomoeopathy : covering the true life of Cesare Mattei and properly transcripted Empirical Formulas & Secret Pharmacy of Electrohomoeopathy, incl. Medicinal Plants Used by Cesare Mattei.

Contributors-Prof. Raffaele Pezzani, University of Padova, Italy, Dr. Fabio R. Ambrosi, University of Sapienza, Rome, Italy, Prof. El Akrem Hayouni, University of Manouba, Tunisia, Allesandro Rapparini, Vice Pres., Archivio Museo Cesare Mattei, Bologna, Italy, Prof. Peter Morrell, Formerly Honorary Research Associate, History of Medicine, Staffordshire University, U.K., Dr. Terry Mitchell, Alchemist & Director, Phylak GmbH, U.K., Willow Morningsky, Spagyrist & Psychologist, Southern Oregon University, Ashland, Oregon, U.S.A. etc.

CONTENTS: Introduction, Dedication, Note to the Readers, Acknowledgements, Alchemist's Prayer, Preface, The Castle of Love, The Mystery Unveiled, Emerald Tablet of Cesare Mattei, Mysticism & Romance of Cesare Mattei, Electro Homoeopathy Pharmacology, Medicinal Plants Used by Cesare Mattei, Glossary of Pharmacological Terms, Bibliography

For Further Information and Ordering:
Originals/Low Price Publications
A-6, Second Floor, Nimri Commercial Centre,
Ashok Vihar Phase-4, Delhi - 110 052 (India)
Tel.: +91 11 2730 2453 Fax: 011 4706 1936
Mobile: 98100-12366
Website: www.Lppindia.com,
e-mail: info@Lppindia.com
info@Lbopub.com